COLOUR THERAPY WORKBOOK

COLOUR THERAPY WORKBOOK

The classic guide from the pioneer of colour healing

Theo Gimbel

Thorsons

Thorsons
An Imprint of HarperCollins*Publishers*
77–85 Fulham Palace Road,
Hammersmith, London W6 8JB

The Thorsons website address is: www.thorsons.com

and *Thorsons*
are trademarks of HarperCollins*Publishers* Ltd

First published by Element Books 1993
This edition published by Thorsons 2002

10 9 8 7 6 5 4 3 2 1

© Theo Gimbel 1993, 2002

Theo Gimbel asserts the moral right to be
identified as the author of this work

A catalogue record of this book is
available from the British Library

ISBN 0 00 714540 3

Printed and bound in Great Britain by
Scotprint, Haddington, East Lothian

Contents

Acknowledgements

I would like to thank Carmel Dunleavy-Gimbel for her good advice and help in all directions of the work in hand, and also Rita Legg, who is always ready to correct and type thousands of words and rephrase some of the sentences slightly more succinctly!

Introduction

Colour therapy harnesses the energies of light and the colours of the spectrum to help a wide variety of health problems and to allow us to harmonize with our natural rhythms and energies, and generally to become more balanced. It does this by locating and then correcting colour imbalances in the aura, the energy field surrounding the body.

All true therapies acknowledge that the five senses are gateways to healing. Sight is a gateway to colour healing; hearing is a gateway for music therapy; touch lends itself to massage; smell to aromatherapy; and taste to our diet. Remember, we are what we eat and our diet plays a very important part in the healing process.

To acknowledge our senses is important because in colour therapy we treat a person as a whole, comprising body, mind and spirit. Each of these three aspects contains colour, which becomes finer and more ethereal as it reaches into the spirit.

As humanity evolves, awareness and consciousness change. Perhaps it is because of this evolutionary change that there are now many different schools of colour therapy, each teaching a slightly different technique but all ultimately reaching towards the same goal.

This book will introduce you to the history and application of colour therapy, and in particular to the methods I have developed since 1956. To give you a taste of this, I would like to describe briefly a typical colour healing session.

A Colour Healing Session

First the patient is made welcome. A 'stage report' is compiled. This is a record of the patient's past illnesses, treatment received, operations, drugs, etc. The patient's present problem is recorded and they are invited to say why they chose colour therapy as a method of treatment.

We emphasize to each new patient that colour therapy is *complementary to qualified medical treatment* and that they must always follow their medical doctor's advice.

A 'spine chart' is then compiled (*see page 64*). This is a chart of the human spine that we ask the patient to sign on the back. Their signature acts as a 'witness' because it contains their energy, and it is this energy that we are then able to pick up.

We then dowse out each individual vertebra using a dowsing technique described on page 63. Wherever there is a reaction, the relevant vertebra on the spine chart is marked with a cross. This chart is then interpreted and the appropriate colours for therapy are selected.

The patient puts on a white robe (to prevent colour distortion) and sits comfortably in the therapy room. The selected colour plates (made of stained glass) are fitted into the colour therapy instrument (*see page 60*).

The instrument is then started. During the $19^3/_4$-minute session relaxing music is played. The treatment colour, with its complementary colour, is beamed at the patient in a fixed cycle which is timed by an electronic timer. The patient may talk or sleep during the session.

After the session, the patient is asked how they feel. Do they feel the colours inside their body? Do they feel an increased sense of well-being or any side effects?

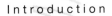

Finally, a series of seven colour therapy treatments is advised, one per week, to give the patient's body time to adjust and respond.

Objectivity and Intuition

Without exception, anyone who wishes to learn colour therapy must learn to be objective; to let go of all preconceived ideas and to be, at least when working on behalf of others, a neutral person with an ear to listen and an eye to see rather than to spend most of the time talking and being inquisitive.

Maturity is not necessarily linked to age and intelligence, but to a true will to observe and have only the patient's interest at heart. This in itself will open up the practitioner to respond, often in quite surprising ways. They may suddenly know exactly the right thing to do for the patient and the correct way of applying it. This knowledge comes from intuition and it is only by listening that we will hear and know.

Chapter 1

What is Colour Therapy?

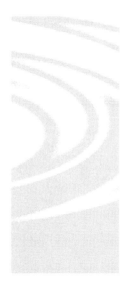

... and darkness was upon the face of the deep. And the Spirit of God moved upon the face of the waters.

And God said, Let there be light: and there was light.

Genesis 1:2–3

Thus darkness and light began the sacred dance of creation and out of their dance were born all the colours of the rainbow. Each colour holds within itself its opposite complementary colour. You can experience this for yourself by doing the following exercise.

Practical Exercise

Take a white sheet of paper, not smaller than one square foot (77 square cm). In the middle place a clear-coloured six-inch diameter square or circle or any other shape that you wish.

Look at this colour for about 15 seconds.

Now turn over the paper quickly and look at the blank side. You will find, after a short while, that its complementary colour will appear. It will be very bright, almost like a light. The quality of this colour will be like the colours found in the aura or electromagnetic field that surrounds a stone, plant, animal or human being.

Colour and the Electromagnetic Spectrum

Colour is a part of the electromagnetic spectrum. Long before it appears as the visible part of this spectrum, we find cosmic frequencies which have such a fast vibrational frequency that they cannot be measured. These rays are in the realm of darkness. Light can be measured against darkness and has a speed of 180,000 miles per second. When this slows down, we reach the point where colour begins. This starts with ultra-violet and continues with the colours of the spectrum. The slowing down of this spectrum after it goes beyond infra-red brings us sounds which are beyond human hearing. This occurs at about 22,000 cycles per second (cps). Sound then slows to a very slow beat that can decompose architectural structures. Finally, it will stand still at zero (0) and can be seen as static form (*see Figure 1.1*).

Apart from the cosmic rays, all of the invisible part of the electromagnetic spectrum is used by science or medicine, sometimes resulting in harmful side effects. The visible part of the spectrum, namely the eight colours (*see page 5*), each one with its own vibrational frequency, is thought to have no effect upon us. Through research which I have carried out, as have others in this field, such as Max Lüscher, Faber Birren and Roland Hunt to name but a few, it has been shown that this is untrue. One simple example is the effect that red and blue light have on blood pressure. It has been proven that red light raises blood pressure whereas blue light lowers it.

All living things, including the human race, have their own vibrational frequency. Each muscle, bone and organ of the human body

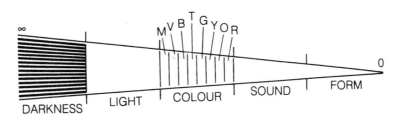

Figure 1.1: The electromagnetic spectrum.

vibrates to its own frequency and it is these frequencies that produce the electromagnetic field surrounding us. This is also known as the aura. This electromagnetic field or aura contains all the colours of the spectrum and they are constantly changing in volume, shade and density according to our state of health or mood.

According to Rudolf Steiner, Annie Besant and G. I. Gurdjieff, a human being is composed of an ego and an astral, an etheric and a physical body. Steiner defines the ego as the consciousness and individuality of a person that is linked to the higher or true spiritual self. It is from here that our true inspiration comes. The astral body (also known as the psyche or soul) is that part of us which feels emotion and harmony and through which we experience peace and tranquillity. The etheric body houses the life force that feeds the physical body, keeping its energies in harmony and balance. It is these energies that can obey both our soul and our ego. Indeed, if we think positively about ourselves it makes us feel better, allowing our soul to experience harmony. If we were able to live constantly in this state, dis-ease would be eradicated.

Through this teaching, Steiner creates for us a picture of man as a five-fold being:

○ the spirit, self, God, being (the part of creation where we would find the angelic world);
○ the ego, personality, mental body, which is already linked to our thought patterns;
○ the astral, soul, feeling, emotional body (that part of us where we can experience joy, happiness, fear, hate, etc.);
○ the etheric, life force, metabolic body (the area where energy is extracted from the food we eat);
○ the physical body.

Further energies exist above the spirit self and below the physical body, but these can only be experienced through the growth of consciousness. All of these are represented in the electromagnetic field or aura that surrounds us.

If any part of our being, any organ, muscle, gland or bone, is out of harmony, then the frequency of its vibration changes and disease follows. This also brings about a change in the colours which surround us in our aura.

What then is colour therapy? Colour therapy is using the vibrational frequency of the colours of the spectrum to correct imbalance or disharmony in the human body.

The Eight Major Colours

Time as we know it is measured by the Earth's circulatory journey around the sun. We can start at any time of the day or night to look at the colours which play around the Earth as the sun circles the planet. Let us begin at the early morning hour when most of us are still asleep (see Figure 1.2).

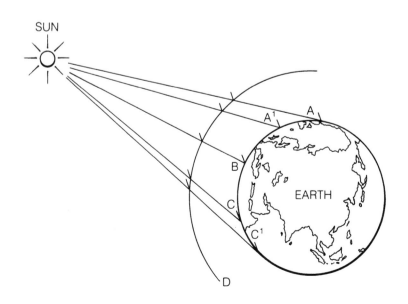

Figure 1.2: The light of the sun which comes down to the earth at dawn.
A Very shallow and casts long shadows.
A¹ These shadows quickly become shorter.
At mid-day the shadows become very short.
The colours of the general atmosphere are coming out of the violet–blue gradually into the greens (B).
C Early evening turns into yellows, oranges.
C¹ The day ends with red before the sun sinks on the horizon.
D This is the air cloak round this planet that makes the light visible.

5

It is 1 a.m. and a very fine, deep colour emerges from the apparent darkness. It is the colour purple. For the next two hours this royal colour prevails, changing imperceptibly towards violet as the hour of 3 a.m. approaches. This is the night colour that surrounds us in sleep. Its very high vibration endows us with healing qualities needed in preparation for the coming day. Many children choose to be born at this hour because it is the hour of renewal. It is also the hour during which many souls choose to return to the world from which they originally manifested.

Gradually, violet turns into blue as we approach the hour of dawn. This varies between 5 and 7 a.m., depending upon the time of year. The blue changes into turquoise and the freshness of this colour takes over the day. At 9 a.m. turquoise changes into a peacock green, spreading over the morning hours to 11 a.m. when a pure green emerges. This stays with us until the beginning of the afternoon. At 1 p.m. the atmosphere is filled with an apple green with a hint of yellow. Towards 3 p.m. the true yellow begins, changing into orange at about 5 p.m. At this time people tend to relax. The worker goes home and joins their family or companions. It is the hour to be social. By 7 p.m. evening has come and in the summer months the sun is sinking, toning the evening sky with red before night falls. Red is the colour of strength and of life. Around 9 p.m., as the evening draws to a close, this red turns into a deep mauve. Night has started and as we sleep, the beautiful colour of magenta takes us through the midnight hours from 11 p.m. to 1 a.m.

Some people may see these changes but most people cannot. To see them for yourself, take a photograph of a garden or landscape in the morning. Two hours later take another photograph of the same scene. Repeat this throughout the day. You will find that each picture has a different colour overlaying the scene. The photograph taken in the early morning will be much bluer and in the afternoon much yellower.

In the summer, go into the country, away from all the street lights, and look up into the clear sky. You will see that the stars are set against a deep mauve–magenta–purple heaven. The colours are so deep that our eyes perceive them as black, but I assure you that they are not.

One thing which may have occurred to you is that the six night hours between 9 p.m. and 3 a.m. display colours which are very closely linked in their hues, giving the impression that the colour changes are much slower. During the morning and evening the colour changes are quicker. This, of course, has an effect on those who work on night shifts out in the open.

Looking at the colours which appear through the day and night and the seasons of the year, we can see that each colour has an individuality and yet remains in harmony with the whole rainbow. Each colour has its own particular place. The orange stands between red and yellow. The green between yellow and turquoise. The blue between violet and turquoise and the red between magenta and orange.

Thus we have come full circle, or perhaps it is more correct to say that we have covered a first spiral, which has no beginning and no end. It descends into even stronger, darker colours and ascends into ever lighter shades.

Colour therapists begin to experience these perceptions as they become more aware of colour, its energy, its meaning and how it can be used to help mankind.

Figure 1.3

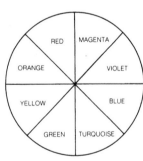

Chapter 2

A History of Colour Therapy

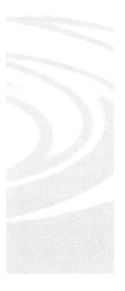

The old order changes, yielding place to new
And God fulfils himself in many ways
Lest one good custom should corrupt the world ...

Alfred Lord Tennyson, Morte D'Arthur

Anthropologists have reported that prehistoric man was unable to see colour. This faculty developed later on and is still developing today. More people are now born with the ability to see the colours in the aura.

Atlantis and Egypt

It is believed that in Atlantean times colour was used for healing. According to Frank Alpen in his book *Exploring Atlantis*, the Atlanteans built healing temples. These were circular in shape and around the circumference were individual healing rooms. When a person entered these rooms, a crystal door closed behind them. This was then energized to the frequency of the colour required. The ceiling of the main temple was domed and made of interlocking crystals. When the light shone through these crystals it formed patterns of colour and vibrations. Crystals and colour were used not only for physical ailments but also for the healing of relationships, and of emotional and mental imbalances. With colour, the Atlanteans also used geometric forms believing these to be as important.

Similarly, archaeologists have discovered that Egyptian temples contained rooms which were constructed to allow the dissipation of the rays of the sun into the colours of the spectrum. They used coloured paints for their temple drawings and their hieroglyphics were equally beautiful in colour. These temples were used not only for worship but also for healing. It is believed that the sick were colour diagnosed and then put into one of the rooms surrounding the temple, which radiated the colour prescribed. This appears to follow closely the colour healing methods of the Atlanteans.

Again like the Atlanteans, the ancient Egyptians used gems in colour treatment. They proclaimed that gems are pure and contain concentrated colour and therefore have the maximum effect upon the body. They would grind up gemstones and administer the powder to the patient. This follows the same principle as Ayurvedic medicine.

The Egyptians also used solarized water in healing. This is a treatment in which water is infused with the vibrational frequency of a prescribed colour (by shining full-spectrum light through a glass of spring water under a given colour) and then drunk in small doses over a set period of time – and it is still used today.

The costumes worn by the Egyptian people were made of natural colours, but the priests' robes were adorned with quantities of blue and gold. How dyes and bleaches were made were temple secrets. Writing, measuring, counting and weighing, as well as correctly melting metals, were skills only taught to the initiated priests.

Colour Pigments Used in Ancient Egypt

1 TO BE USED ON GLASS

Dark blue: Cobalt

Light blue and green: Copper/green: iron

Yellow: Antimony and lead mixture

Rose-gold: Gold mixed with small quantity of iron

Red: Copper oxide

Blue: Silver oxide

2 TO BE USED FOR PAINTING (PIGMENT COLOURS)

Except for black, all colours were of mineral origin.

Black: Soot with powdered charcoal. Resin from trees as a fixing agent

White: Chalk or plaster (heated alabaster)

Red: Red ochre; iron oxide

Dark yellow: Yellow ochre derived from hydrated ferric oxide

Light yellow: Sesqui-sulphuret of arsenic covered with beeswax

In Egyptian mythology, the colours of blue, yellow and red were given to their various gods. The Egyptians believed that blue rays were most powerful in the morning and in the spring and ascribed this colour to Thoth. Thoth was worshipped as a moon god and his name was sometimes given to the moon. Yellow was ascribed to Isis and thought to be the most powerful colour at noon and in the summer. Isis was the wife of Osiris and many things are attributed to her, including the civilization of Egypt. This came about through her teachings to women on how to grind corn, spin flax and weave cloth. She was also responsible for teaching men the art of curing disease. Red, believed to be strongest in the afternoon and in autumn, was attributed to Osiris. At first Osiris was worshipped as a nature god embodying the spirit of vegetation that dies with the harvest to be reborn again in the spring. Later on he was worshipped as god of the dead (*New Larousse Encyclopaedia of Mythology*, 1959).

India

From Egypt we come to India, a nation that still uses colour in its healing techniques, as can be seen in Ayurvedic medicine.

Indian philosophy sees man as a being who wears a coat of many colours – colours which are continually changing according to a person's mental, emotional and physical well-being. This coat is composed of seven bodies which interpenetrate each other and constitute the aura or electromagnetic field. The densest of the layers is the actual physical body containing the quintessence of all the aura layers.

Layer 1	The body
Layer 2	The etheric sheath
Layer 3	The astral sheath
Layer 4	The mental sheath
Layer 5	The higher mental sheath
Layer 6	The personality spirit
Layer 7	The higher self
Layer 8	The spirit self

These layers become finer and finer, and after the eighth are commonly not visible, even to those who can see auras. However, there is a sense that picks up unnamed sheaths which reach into galactic space. Man is identified with the creative forces of the universe, which are seen both through the visible colours of the spectrum and the invisible colours not yet manifested upon Earth.

Contained within these bodies are the seven chakras or energy centres (*see page 43*). These are likened to vortices of energy, each of which radiates one of the colours of the spectrum and is associated with one of the endocrine glands in the physical body. Indian physicians worked with these centres and the aura, looking upon them purely as energy which is either in or out of balance. If a person was ill, they looked not at the symptom of the ailment but at the whole being – body, mind and spirit. They looked for imbalances in the energy field and treated them with colour in the form of coloured gemstones or light. Though not yet accepted by the medical profession, this is the basis for colour healing today.

Traditional Colours and Uniforms

Over the centuries, royal houses have adopted certain colours for their costumes and have become known by them. The different colours of traditional dress adopted by different countries are also well known. The colours used in different parts of the globe were largely dependent upon the availability of certain minerals and their oxides. This tradition has almost been made extinct by the fashion world, in which certain colours are mandatory for certain seasons, disregarding the individuality and needs of each man and woman. Many professionals still tend to wear grey and black striped suits and white shirts with white or blue collars because this is supposed to be businesslike. Even people who wear overalls for work usually dress in either green or blue.

As well as blue and grey (the colours of regulation), more traditional business people dress and surround themselves with brown, the colour of commitment. They wear brown suits and sit in brown-panelled offices with brown carpets. The monks and nuns of the order of St Francis wear brown habits, showing that they have committed themselves to their chosen profession and the vows they have taken.

Wearing black, on the other hand, the colour of bereavement in the West, attracts the energies around people and projects an impression of nothingness. The mourner in black makes a statement of being nothing without their loved one. Priests, who also wear black, learn to be open to the energies this colour attracts and are able to cope with the sense of nothingness it creates.

It is also interesting to note that Western women usually wear white on their wedding day. White is the colour of purity and innocence and was traditionally symbolic of the virgin bride and her purity of mind, heart and body.

In earlier times, armies wore red uniforms with beautifully embroidered jackets, epaulettes, sashes and stars. The buttons of the jacket were a gold colour. The higher the rank, the more elaborate the embroidery. The richer the monarch, the more glorious the uniforms. Today, army uniforms are not designed to show the monarch's power. Instead, the khaki and very earthy colours used act as a camouflage to deceive the enemy.

Scottish tartans date back to the times when it was traditional for families to wear their own colours in the clothes they wore, namely the kilt. The design and colour of the tartan identifies the clan, for example, the Campbells or the Stuarts.

Aniline Dyes

In 1856 there was a major chemical discovery. Sir William Perkin made the first synthetic dyestuff through a distillation of coal-tar products. These were called aniline dyes and they revolutionized the dyeing industry.

Mauve (reddish–violet) was the first of the aniline dyes. Magenta, a red–purple, was also first prepared in the mid-nineteenth century.

There is no danger from aniline dyes once the dye has been fixed: only during the process is it poisonous.

Although the advantage of dyeing with aniline is that the colours will not fade, unfortunately they are not as beautiful and alive as natural colours. An experienced eye can easily detect the difference.

Colour Filters

What people fail to realize is that the colour of the clothes we wear acts as a colour filter which is absorbed by our body. If we are able to become aware and tune into our body, we will know which colour we need to wear to create health and harmony in our whole being.

It is important to realize that colours used for clothes can be both a pigment colour and at the same time a colour filter. This fact plays a very important part in colour therapy and will be enlarged upon in Chapter 3.

Colour in the Christian Era

Stained Glass

In the fourth and fifth centuries, the start of the Byzantine era, art followed a set tradition. In the mosaics and the stained-glass windows of churches and cathedrals, blue represented the heavens and red the royal ruler, either the king or emperor. Maria (mother Mary) was represented as the Queen of Heaven in a blue cloak and a red dress, signifying her special task for this world, which is carried out with love. Up to the seventeenth century the colours used for church windows show that a clear pattern was followed, laid down from an older tradition. At the end of the seventeenth century, a gradual change began. This started with paintings and was followed by the colours used in church windows.

The colours in the stained-glass windows of gothic cathedrals exhibit a special kind of light. The stained glass used in such cathedrals or churches was very carefully made by craftsmen who knew that the full colours could only be achieved through very pure oxides such as gold, silver and copper.

In 1947, Chagall, the great Jewish artist, was persuaded by a Christian priest to design and make the stained-glass windows for Stephans Kirche in Mainz. He asked him to do it in order to make a new link between the Christian Germans and the Jews after the fall of Hitler. Chagall was a deeply religious man with a great depth of spiritual knowledge. He knew how to use colour to express spiritual depth through stained glass and these windows were his last work. He died before they were completed.

Other famous modern stained-glass windows are those of the Goetheanum in Dornach, Switzerland, which were designed by Rudolf Steiner. The Goetheanum is the centre for the study of all human arts and links these to the divinity and spiritual path of mankind. Steiner's teachings are built upon those of Goethe. Each window is made out of 2.5 cm (1 in) thick pure blue, green, rose and red plate glass. Each plate is more than 2 square metres (21 square ft) and four of these plates of glass are mounted on top of each other, making a window of 8 metres (26 ft) high, 2 metres (6 ft) wide. The designs are ground out of this glass so that the very thin colours which are left are the light part of the designs. These windows affect a person greatly because the designs and colours act as a medium for meditation. Each colour is absorbed by the person and induces a particular state of consciousness according to the particular colour.

Blue   Relaxation and peace
Green   Balance and cleansing
Violet   Dignity and self-respect
Rose   Spiritual love

Many stained-glass windows are designed with a New Age consciousness, a state of mind that has come about through the path of meditation, which has only become generally known about since the end of the Second World War.

Colour Pioneers

J. W. Goethe, in his work *Die Farben Lehre*, published in 1810 and translated incorrectly as 'The Theory of Colour' instead of 'The Teachings of Colour', showed how colours are the children of light and darkness.

Sir Isaac Newton (1642–1727) discovered that when daylight entered the dark room in which he was working, the colours of the spectrum appeared. From this discovery, he carried out a scientific appraisal of colour. Sir Isaac Newton and Goethe complement each other in their findings. Newton is very scientific and factual in his observations whereas Goethe gives the psychological, soul experience of colour. J. M. W. Turner, the famous painter, used Goethe's work extensively for his pictures.

More recent writers and explorers in colour therapy include Babbitt, Ousley, Roland Hunt, Dinshah, Faber Birren, Proskauer and Steiner. Steiner also wrote about the use of colour in healing. The Camphill schools, founded by Dr Karl König, and the colour awareness techniques used in all the Rudolf Steiner schools are due to Steiner's influence.

Professor Ronald Gregory of Bristol University was one of the first people to relate colour to psychology. I remember in the 1950s when I mentioned to educational psychologists the important part colour should play in their work, their reactions implied that this was nonsense and in no way were colour and psychology connected. Professor Max Lüscher has proved beyond doubt that colour and the psyche are linked and that colour can help the personality. Testing both individuals and groups of people over many years, he discovered that when people see a colour they have a particular personal reaction. However, he also found that there is a general objective reaction. His work on 'personality' was built on these discoveries.

Out of these early explorations has come what is today accepted as colour therapy.

In 1956, I myself started in a very primitive way to experiment with colour. Through this I realized that there is also a form element connected to colour. Blue, for instance, has a different energy and meaning when it is contained in a circle from when it is contained in a square or triangle. These findings also apply to the remaining colours of the spectrum. We will go into more detail on this in the next chapter.

Chapter 3

What Colour Can Do for You

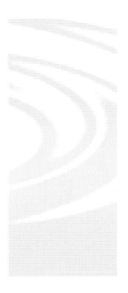

'I am in the right place, at the right time, for the right purpose.'

Anonymous

Colour is a doorway that leads deep into the mind and soul. It has the ability to affect all living things both consciously and unconsciously.

Light splits itself up into all the colours of the rainbow when it reaches the area between ultra-violet and infra-red on the electro-magnetic spectrum. When the frequencies of this spectrum slow down to ultra-violet, the human eye starts to perceive the first rays of magenta, often mistaken for pink. Then violet, blue, turquoise, green, yellow, orange and red appear. After red, the rays again become invisible as they sink into infra-red.

The human body is light-sensitive, allowing colour to be absorbed through its cell structure as well as through the eyes. This means that blind people are equally receptive to colour.

The Five Senses and the Elements

Our five so-called 'normal' senses consist of sight, hearing, taste, smell and touch. Each is connected to an element. Sight is connected to the element of fire; hearing is connected to the element of air; taste is connected to the element of water; and smell is connected to the element of earth. The fifth sense, touch, is connected to the etheric energy. It took many years of research before this energy was accepted as being vital to life. It surrounds all living matter and sensitive people can sense this energy around crystals, stones plants and humans.

Everyone, unless blind, can see the physical body with their eyes, but the etheric energy and aura are experienced through our higher senses. Steiner speaks of 12 senses – which leaves us with seven above the normal five. As our awareness grows, we are able to develop these and 'see' what to many remains unseen.

We will look at this in more detail in the next chapter. First, let us examine the energies each colour transmits and some of the ways in which they can be used in healing. Even though it is possible for people to treat themselves with colour, it is always more beneficial to attend a qualified practitioner.

The Colour Energies and Chakras

Base: Red
A beautiful clear mid-red, not leaning towards either orange or deep purple

Meaning   Strength, energy, vitality, life, sexuality, warning, power, alertness, contraction

Therapeutic use   Low blood pressure, lack of energy, impotence, inactivity, drowsiness

Sacral: Orange

A joyful, cheerful colour lifting out of the red towards yellow

Meaning   Happiness, dance, joy, independence, carelessness, uplift

Therapeutic use   Antidepressant, also for low blood pressure when red is too powerful

Solar Plexus: Yellow

The colour nearest to the light

Meaning   Detachment, intellect, thinking, judgement, criticism

Therapeutic use   Rheumatism, arthritis, controlling calcium, regaining objectivity

Heart: Green

The colour of nature and the plant kingdom

Meaning   Harmony, balance, stability, neutrality

Therapeutic use   Cleansing, purifying, cancer, enhancing thoughts and emotions

Thymus: Turquoise

A clear, fresh morning colour

Meaning   Purity, immunity, calmness

Therapeutic use   Anti-inflammatory, AIDS (HIV), nervous tension

Thyroid: Blue

The colour of the sky and sea, receding into the distance

Meaning   Relaxation, sleep, peace, expansion

Therapeutic use   High blood pressure, stress, asthma, migraine

Pituitary: Violet

An uplifting, spiritual colour

Meaning   Dignity, divinity, honour, value, hope

Therapeutic use   Hopelessness, lack of self-respect, loss of self-appreciation, building personality

Pineal: Magenta

A colour of the highest order

Meaning   Selflessness, meditation, perfection, release

Therapeutic use   Changes, freedom, to let go of old habits no longer applicable, the final transition into spirit at the correct time

White

The colour that contains all colours

Meaning   Untouched, innocence, isolation, wisdom, representing the priest

Therapeutic use   Total neutrality, absolute clarity, truth

Black

The unfathomable depth, holding all colours which are earthbound, experience

Meaning   Attraction, humility, negativity, knowledge personified, science

Therapeutic use   Not applied in colour therapy

Grey

A colour that denies being a colour

Meaning   Service, dedication

Therapeutic use   Pride, haughtiness (rarely if ever used)

Brown

The colour of the earth, death

Meaning   Sacrifice, dedication, commitment

Therapeutic use   Only applied in colour therapy to those who are completely selfish, not making any contribution to anything or anybody. (In this case the colour should be worn in a dress or suit)

Complementary Colours

Figure 3.1: This chart shows the eight main colours of the spectrum and their complementary colour.

Each of these colours has a complementary colour. Both the colour and its complementary are used in colour therapy (*see pages 59–60*). To find the complementary colour, see Figure 3.1.

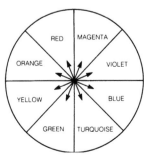

The Eyes and Colour

Colours always work in complementary ways. This is also true of our eyes. When the rods and cones in the retina focus on one single colour, they will naturally produce the complementary colour. People are usually unaware of this because they do not allow time to experience this change. During this change, our eyes go into contraction and expansion, causing movement to the whole cell structure. As well as activating the rods and cones, we activate the muscles of the iris. This experience should keep the eyes healthy and strong. Why then are we faced today with so many eye problems, which are diagnosed by the optician as normal deterioration? About 200 years ago, eye problems of today's magnitude were unknown. This is partly due to the fact that in our present age, more people read, write, drive, use computers and watch television.

Colour is influential in the focusing of the eye. Blue focuses in front of the retina, red behind the retina and green on the retina. Blue light, which is also daylight, is the kindest light for the human eye. Green light breaks down all biochemical cells in their early stages, so it can be very helpful as a complementary therapy in healing cancer. Via the eyes, relayed to the pituitary gland, it directs the body and, under doctor's supervision, can be very successful. Pregnant women need to be careful, however, with VDUs.

Since 1956, the Hygeia College of Colour Therapy has conducted research into the colour reactions of the eyes. This has resulted in the production of the eye strengthening chart (*see Figure 3.2*).

The chart displays a red octagon and a blue octagon on a white background to prompt a reaction when the eye moves from the red to the blue and then to the central white, thus experiencing the appearance of the complementary colour as a luminous glowing light. The red causes a contraction of the eye cells and the blue makes them expand. Thus, the eye 'breathes' in and out. The success of the eye strengthening chart has been outstanding.

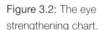

Figure 3.2: The eye strengthening chart.

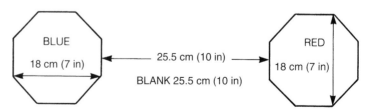

BLUE
18 cm (7 in)
25.5 cm (10 in)
BLANK 25.5 cm (10 in)
RED
18 cm (7 in)

Practical Exercise

Stand the eye strengthening chart up at eye level under good day-light conditions (near a window in bad weather or winter).

Let your eyes rest on the blue and 'soak in' this colour until a luminous area appears around the octagon shape and the colour of the shape itself begins to change.

Then look at the white middle until a luminous, glowing light appears.

Let this fade and then rest your eyes on the red octagon again for a while until the same glow and change of colour appears.

Return to the white centre and now see the whole glow appear again. Look for as long as it takes for this to fade out gradually.

Then return to the blue and repeat this four to seven times, finishing up with the blue, not the red.

Do this once or twice daily.

Colour and Health

The importance of colour in the maintenance of health can no longer be brushed aside. Evidence has shown that it is a very significant factor. Colour, like sound and radio waves, is an energy, but on a much higher frequency. It can therefore treat conditions which are caused by very fine imbalances in the body. It is completely safe and has no known side effects. Students studying colour soon realize how very integrated the spectrum is and learn to appreciate its beneficial effect upon the emotional and mental aspects of a person. This is important, for the mind affects the body, just as the body affects the mind.

Colour Dressing for Health

When you are dressing to go out, there are several points you should try to take into account:

1   The colour
2   Combining colours (the colours you can wear over or underneath each other to enhance your health)
3   The type of material

Let us look at the colours in the sequence of the spectrum.

Red stands for energy. Wearing red can help raise low blood pressure and combat infertility.
Orange brings joy. Wearing orange can lift the spirits.
Yellow causes detachment. Wearing yellow can help rheumatism and arthritis.
Violet induces dignity. Wearing violet enhances self-respect and uplifts the soul.
Blue causes relaxation. Wearing blue overcomes stress, induces a feeling of ease and can help lower blood pressure.
Turquoise brings a tranquillizing energy. Wearing turquoise has a purifying effect and is good for immunity.

These two trios of energy – red, orange and yellow and violet, blue and turquoise – are also complementary to each other.

In Figure 3.3 each of the three pairs of complementary colours has been bracketed together: blue and orange, red and turquoise, violet and yellow. The two triangles represent the first trio, red, orange and yellow ascending, and the second trio, violet, blue and turquoise descending.

Let us now mix turquoise and yellow. *Green* has arisen out of this pairing and is the balance. Wearing green is cleansing and purifying. It can help in the treatment of cancer.

Indigo and navy blue induce deep relaxation and reduce tension. Wearing indigo and navy blue can very quickly reduce or even dissolve pain which is caused by stress and general tension.

Figure 3.3

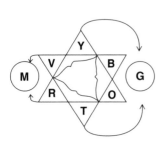

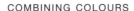

COMBINING COLOURS

What colours can we successfully combine and which should we avoid when we dress to increase our well-being or support our health?

First, we should try to wear white or a compatible colour of under-wear. White combines with all colours and is therefore the easiest colour to recommend for all the eight colours or shades of these.

When we need *red* we can have white, orange or yellow over or under it.

When *orange* is the colour we need, yellow is acceptable but not red.

With *yellow* we can use white but no other colours as these would distort the very sensitive yellow.

Violet should not be worn with blue as it will change the energy to that of indigo. So white is all we can use.

When we use *violet* together with *magenta* we create a purple which will significantly alter both these colours.

Purple can be worn with blue, but be aware it will usually revert to an indigo.

Blue can be worn with turquoise, but makes a more significant impact; white is therefore really the only colour that will combine with blue.

Turquoise with green will alter the turquoise quite considerably and tends to create a peacock green; therefore, again this should be avoided.

Green is a strong colour and can cope with turquoise if this is a soft pastel shade. Otherwise just use white. With yellow it tends to become apple green and changes its energy.

Magenta is a very sensitive colour and quickly changes when used with violet or red. Therefore white remains, as always, the most neutral colour in combination.

For the best results wear your 'health dress' and the complementary colour for a third of the time.

FABRICS

We can describe a human being as having four energy patterns.

1   The God or spirit energy
2   The soul or being energy
3   The life force energy
4   The physical, visible energy

To these four main aspects we can allocate four natural fabrics as follows.

Silk natural to the spirit
Cotton to the soul
Linen to the life force or etheric energy
Wool to the body, the 'coach' that allows us to travel on this solid
     planet

Visualization

We could say that all dis-ease has a mental origin unless it is caused by an accident. Even then, the very first thoughts which follow that accident are important. Basically, there are two types of people: those who succumb to negative, fearful images and those who rise above them and affirm that they will get better. These people can see beyond the momentary problem. Most powerful in all situations is an inner picture which ends with a solution to the problem. This is known as visualization.

The making of images starts by relating words or phrases to a picture which is made up of past memories. Very often it also hinges on aromas. (The sense of smell is a very powerful agent and should only be introduced into a therapy by a qualified therapist.)

Children pick up positive and negative images very quickly. By the age of three, they love to hear stories which enable them to make their own images. Even the horrible witch and the nasty giant are only as bad and horrible as the child can make them out of past experiential memory.

The visual memory of children is enormous. Because they do not read or write they are much more observant and store in their minds what we adults look up in encyclopaedias. They quickly form images out of words, and from descriptions in tales and stories they make pictures in their minds, remember pictures and learn to 'dream visualize' their personal scenes. Television and films, however, take away this creativity and damage this capacity. As we mature, we find that the images we make are richer and more complete. We can use these to help ourselves over many difficulties and increase our own health and well-being. In all of my work since 1967, we have used visualization. It is a technique that goes back to Steiner, who introduced it into meditation.

In the visualization process we form positive images of colours and pictures which help us to change the dis-harmony in our body to harmony. Relate images to your own needs, swim with the river and use its current as a means to approach the current stage in which you find yourself. Cooperate with the forces which surround you, even if at present you are unable to accept them all. Be awake, and at every turn in the river's course, look to see if there is something which you can use to help yourself. Those who swim against the river's flow rarely win. In extreme situations, anchor the mind onto a meaningful familiar image, mantra, prayer or story. It will lead you out of the problems into a new stream of energy which perhaps you could not recognize before.

At difficult times, also remember that what the inner self does while the outer self complies with external circumstances always leads to a new capacity. We can remain strong in our own inner being and do not have to conform as long as we do not offend or injure anyone or anything.

Breathing in Colours

S.K., one of our patients, came complaining of sleeplessness. This had started after an accident two and a half years ago in which she had sustained a knee injury. Since that time her knee had not been free from pain and she had difficulty in bending it. On examination, I noticed that it was very badly scarred and unusually warm to the touch. This suggested that inflammation was still present.

I made a chart for her (*see Chapter 5*) and the diagnostic colour that it revealed was turquoise. I instructed her to breathe in turquoise and to breathe out red for at least five minutes each night before she went to sleep. When I saw her the following week, she reported that she had followed my instructions and had had four nights' uninterrupted sleep. She continued with this exercise on my instructions: her disturbed nights gradually diminishing and the swelling and pain in her knee subsided.

Asthma

Many people suffer from asthma. This can have many causes, but the main symptom is difficulty in breathing caused by spasms of the smooth muscles that lie in the walls of the smaller bronchi and bronchioles causing the passage ways to partially close.

A therapy very conducive to easing an attack is blue light because blue light expands all biochemical structures. (When using coloured lights as a therapy, it is important that they have dimmer switches so that they can gradually be turned on and off.) (Remember, if you are treating yourself with colour you should only wear white, otherwise the colour of the clothes you wear acts as a coloured filter and the colour the body absorbs is a combination of the light and your clothes.)

Some asthma attacks are known to have an underlying rhythm. Some occur at night, others in the early morning or late afternoon. Try and discern which pattern your attacks follow and have a blue light available so that when an attack starts you can switch this light on and gradually increase its intensity.

To reduce an attack successfully you should wear white or blue. Asthma sufferers should not wear red or black. Red cloth and, even more powerfully, red light always contracts all biochemical cells exposed to it; blue cloth and blue light expand cells. They are therefore very helpful for migraine, stress, high blood pressure and general respiratory problems as well as asthma.

Autism

Colour therapy can be a direct or indirect treatment, and therefore it is very suitable in helping autistic children. If possible, they should be treated as soon as the condition has been diagnosed.

The treatment works on the principle that because colour has a very high vibrational frequency, it has a very gentle effect upon such children. We can help them with this therapy but cannot always promise a complete cure. Fringe influences, such as their living environment, have to be taken into account, and these can either support or disrupt the treatment.

In my experience, all autistic children can speak. However, because they have developed a greatly increased level of consciousness at an early age, they suffer from a high degree of shyness. This shyness prevents them from talking because they are frightened that they will make a mistake which would cause them a great deal of pain. Colour can be used to harmonize their extremely high perception levels and produce an invisible protective field around them.

The treatment is known to be a slow process and patience has to be exercised. I feel that it is important to meet the parents with the child. At this meeting we explain how colour therapy works. The first consultation, which includes treatment, usually lasts for one and a half to two hours. This is then followed by monthly treatments, usually over a period of two to four years.

High and Low Blood Pressure

Another complaint that can be alleviated with colour is high or low blood pressure. Blood pressure is the pressure exerted by blood on the wall of a blood vessel. It is generated by cardiac output, which is determined by the rate and force of the heartbeat and the resistance to the flow of blood through the vessels. An increase in the heart rate and an increase in resistance increases blood pressure. The reverse applies for low blood pressure.

If you are suffering from low blood pressure, the colour to use is red. Again, this can be applied with the aid of a red bulb or through red clothing. Another way in which you can treat yourself is to obtain a full-length piece of cotton or silk dyed (with a natural dye) to the colour required. Lie under this in a bright sunny room, either dressed in white or, if it is in the privacy of your own home, naked, for 20 minutes each day.

If you suffer from high blood pressure the same procedure applies, except that you would use blue instead of red.

Visualization for Asthma and Claustrophobia Sufferers

It is a cloudy grey day and you are in a small boat on a canal. The banks have become quite steep and as you look ahead, a lock comes into view. On either side of the boat are very dark walls. As you drive or row into the lock, the sluice gates close behind you and for a moment you find yourself in a dark space. There is so little light and you feel that there is so little hope. You look up to the sky and the sky looks down upon you. The sound of rushing water meets your ears and the panic of being enclosed, shut in, is slightly eased. The feeling of hope unlocks a little of the anxiety. The boat is lifted up as the water rises and the hope of freedom grows. The dark walls of the lock become less visible as you rise to the new level of the canal. Just as the upper lock is beginning to open, the clouds part and the sun shines on to the new level of water to which you have risen. The upper lock gates are now fully open and your boat sails into the clear, free stretch of the canal. The green grass on either side of the canal allows you to change your feelings. You choose the feeling of freedom created by the open free space. This holds a promise for the future. The blue sky shines down on this scene. You have made it.

Starting this visualization will gradually evoke a mental, emotional reaction as you visualize the last rays of light as you drive into the darkness of the lock. The whole picture will become one event out of time and space. When you are next in a situation which has previously caused you problems, take the whole visualization into yourself and all the necessary images will immediately arise: canal journey, boat, lock, darkness, clouds, rush of water, rising water level, sunshine, upper lock gates open, freedom ahead.

This can finally be summed up as:

Darkness is followed by light.
Darkness equals light.
Light follows darkness.

In this way you have overcome the usual fear because you are able to be your own conductor, director of your health. Your thoughts and emotions now control your metabolic and physical reactions so that your cell structure does not have to contract any more. It behaves in a healthy way.

This visualization was written for Clifford S., a patient who suffered with asthma.

Other Disorders

Living in the twenty-first century, with all its haste and problems, creates a lot of stress and tension. If this is not eradicated, it can lead to more serious problems such as cancer. This can be helped with green light, while blue light is excellent against stress. Again you can use a blue bulb or a full-length piece of material (see above).

If you suffer from insomnia, try sleeping in blue sheets, wearing either a blue or white nightdress or pyjamas. Have a blue light burning in the room. This form of treatment is much better than resorting to sleeping tablets. Sleeping tablets have side effects, colour does not.

Depression or lack of energy can be treated with orange. If you suffer from a skin complaint, try using yellow light on it. Yellow is also good for arthritis. If you have cut yourself and it has turned septic, try shining a turquoise light on it. If you have a sore throat, tie a turquoise scarf around it.

These are but a few of the ways in which people can help themselves with colour. If you have a more serious complaint and wish to be treated with colour therapy, do seek the advice of a professionally trained practitioner.

The Golden Ball

To conclude this part of the chapter, I would like to tell the story of how a little girl in Germany used colour to help herself.

Claudia came home from school in tears. When asked what the problem was she said that her classmate had got all the children to 'gang up' on her. She wanted to be friends with her classmate but at this precise moment she hated Claudia.

I told her that hate will only create more hate and that she must learn to love, that no one really hates or is nasty but that people can be got at by things which are making hate or making nastiness. I also told her that sometimes things happen to make us aware that nasty things also have the power to become nice. She listened and then asked me how she could make peace with her schoolfriend.

I told her that she should go into a very quiet place and think of a golden ball and then ask her guardian angel to fill this golden ball with love. After she had done this she should put her friend and herself inside it so that they could both be surrounded by this love and forget the nasty things which had happened.

Claudia went to bed and made her special visualization. When she went to school the next day she had no fear. A few weeks later, I received a letter from Claudia. It read:

Dear Theo,

The golden ball worked wonderfully.

I imagined my schoolfriend and myself in a beautiful desert. We were enveloped by a golden ball in which was mirrored a rainbow.

Yours, Claudia

I had not said anything about a rainbow, but is this not a symbol of peace?

I learnt this method during my time as a prisoner of war in Russia. It works wonders. If children were taught how to do this, violence could be diminished. If schools were open to accept these teachings, I feel that we would be able to help those youngsters who are disturbed or violent.

Colour and Interior Design

The colours we surround ourselves with in everyday life, at work, home or in public, have a subtle yet profound effect on us. If you are considering redecorating your home it is worth thinking about the use of the individual rooms and taking take care over the colour schemes you choose. The table below is based on pure colours as seen in daylight. However, note that paints are rarely pure in colour, as they are often mixed to create slightly different shades. The other trace colours also have a subtle effect on you and you should check these against the chart as well. Often, paints are mixed with white to make them paler. This tones down the effect of the pure colour. For example, pure red has an overstimulating effect and increases blood pressure, whereas pink has a much milder effect. It will increase alertness without exhausting you.

Magenta

Effect: The colour of spiritual fulfilment; good for intuition; induces feelings of wonder, tenderness and completeness

Room: Entrance hall, chapels, lecture theatres; not good for entertainment areas

Violet

Effect: Calming and uplifting; encourages feelings of self-worth, reverence and personal dignity

Room: Chapels, lecture theatres, entrance halls, particularly in hospitals; not recommended for wards and treatment rooms

Blue

Effect: Deeply relaxing; helps lower blood pressure and ease insomnia, nervous conditions and asthma; good for making low ceilings seem higher

Room: Bedrooms, treatment rooms, especially for nervous disorders, offices; not good in entertainment areas

Turquoise

Effect: Refreshing, calming and cleansing; supports the immune system; makes small rooms seem more spacious

Room: Kitchens, treatment rooms, especially where there is the threat of infection, bedrooms, offices; not recommended in children's play areas

Green

Effect: Balancing and neutralizing; encourages balanced judgement but also indecision

Room: Difficult to use without making the room feel flat and empty; suitable for boardrooms and operating theatres

Yellow

Effect: Makes people feel uneasy and detached; encourages judgemental behaviour

Room: Corridors or rooms you do not want people to spend time in

Orange

Effect: Encourages joy, movement and dance; an antidepressant

Room: Entertainment areas, e.g. dining rooms, dance halls; not good for bedrooms or offices

Red

Effect: Colour of strength, power and sexuality; increases blood pressure and makes people feel excited, sensual and domineering; normally overstimulating and overwhelming; makes rooms seem smaller

Room: Activity area; not good for bedrooms or stressful environments

Black

Effect: Emotionally demanding

Room: Not suitable as a dominant colour

White

Effect: Suggests innocence and purity; rejects intrusion

Room: Too stark to use alone; compensate with other colours or plants, ornaments, pictures, etc

Therapeutic Use of Colour in Art and Design

How people experience colour in paintings, posters and everyday objects depends upon their state of well-being. A pretty landscape, yacht or beautifully painted flowers can make a good decorative setting in the so-called 'normal' state of mind. The same picture viewed by a patient in a hospital, surgery or clinic more often than not causes them to feel 'shut out' from it because it tries to give the impression that all is well when inwardly the patient or observer knows that with them all is not well. This then produces an introverted state of mind which can result in the person not being able to communicate with the doctor whom they have come to see. Valuable time can be saved for both patient and doctor when the patient comes into the treatment room with an open and questioning mind.

In a clinical setting it is therefore important that pictures and decor should be chosen to aid communication and treatment. Images which do not depict representational art are of enormous value in helping to restore mental, emotional and physical health.

Healing Colour in Nature

Many of us are stuck in offices all day and unable to benefit from the healing powers of light outside. If you work in an office it is essential that you step outside and walk around the block for at least 10 minutes a day or, even better, stroll through a local park where you can enjoy the colours of nature. This is particularly important if you work in a windowless environment, as you need adequate amounts of full-spectrum light to boost your seratonin levels and, during the day, to suppress the production of melatonin. Too little full-spectrum light can lead to depression, often known as SAD (seasonal affective disorder), as well as other health problems.

It is now possible to install full-spectrum lighting, so if you are worried about getting too little natural lighting, speak to your employer. You will find that most offices are lit with fluorescent tube lighting, which often causes or aggravate stress-related problems, such as headaches, because it flickers constantly. If you are concerned, ask your employer to install full-spectrum lighting or, at the very least, to replace the usual starter in the fluorescent tube with an electronic ballast (*see page 73*). This will override the flicker and stabilize the light. Alternatively, you can buy daylight simulation bulbs from most good electrical shops. You can fit these in desk lamps for a more natural light (*see also Resources on page 123*).

At weekends, make sure you spend at least two or three hours outdoors. Gardening is a particularly good way to do this, for not only will you benefit from the natural light but you will also absorb the healing colour energies from the plants and flowers you are tending. You can plant your garden with different coloured flowers, shrubs and herbs depending on the colours you need for healing (*see list below*).

HEALING FLOWERS AND PLANTS

Plant your garden with the colours that you need for healing or feel drawn to.

Magenta:	Fuchsias
Violet:	Pansies, violets
Blue:	Cornflowers, bluebells, hyacinths
Turquoise:	None known
Green:	Grass, shrubs, trees
Yellow:	Daffodils, primroses, tulips
Orange:	Marigolds
Red:	Roses, tulips

THE HEALING GARDEN

... And there I sat, the window at my left
Counting my bills, examining my tax,
Planning, with intellect, the day's programme
Answering all letters of professional importance –
Being engrossed in business and my post.

Outside, the sky, the trees, my garden call.
My watch, however, tells me: Get on! Work! –
... my concentration starts to slip
Yet silently my garden calls.
Now in my soul there grows a tug of war –
Why do I have to watch the clock?

Whom do I obey? My mind? Or should I let my soul decide?
But now my soul has won.
The pen slips from my hand – and let the phone just ring.

I am away! The door into my garden opens wide
And in a different world I stand.

Out there – the green grass leaves me free to choose.
Shall I sit down and dream? But over there –
A cluster of blue flowers lures me on
To have a closer look. What peace now lets my soul
Relax into this pool of blue.
There is no time, no space, just blue.

And like in dreams a world of beauty
Tells no time – and far away my inner vision
Gives to skies and seas – to warmth and endless ways
Peace of mind which only moments past
Was busy, locked and shut in time.

I turn my eyes and there a patch of orange marigolds
Now look at me as if to say: Come dance with us.
We take you to a place of joy
And make your heart to love us all.

And over in that patch, against the wall,
I now can see the rhododendron shrubs
Their beautiful magenta blossoms say: Let go,
Do change your lifestyle. We renew your thoughts
So that you may easily do your work.

And these ten minutes in my garden healed
My mind and cleared my thoughts
And all, in spite of time, that day was done
So I was proud to slip away from work.

My healing garden does not have to call me now
– I go each day, because my soul is clear.
My garden now does heal me every day
And yet my work gets done with greater ease.

Theophilus Gimbel 24.2.2000

Chapter 4

The Aura and the Chakras

If the light of a thousand suns suddenly arose in the sky, that splendour might be compared to the radiance of the Supreme Spirit. And Arjuna saw in that radiance the whole universe in its variety, standing in a vast unity, in the body of God ...

Bhagavad Gita, Ch. 2, v. 1213; translated by Juan Mas Caro, Penguin Classics

All things that are visible, from stones to plants, animals, human beings, water, fire, air and minerals, contain energy. Generally we are able to weigh, measure or quantify this energy by one method or another.

For many people, this knowledge is sufficient. However, as we enter the twenty-first century, more people are beginning to sense that all objects which are visible also have an invisible counterpart. This invisible energy can be likened to a magnet. Only a few see the force that surrounds a magnet, known as magnetism, but its existence can be proven by showing its power to attract metal objects to it.

In the same way, around all things visible there is an invisible 'cloak', known as the aura or electromagnetic field. The auras around dense matter, such as minerals, have very bright colours. The aura surrounding stones is mainly white with a very fine magenta tint.

Plants have a golden aura, animals a mainly blue one and humans a multi-coloured one.

The aura of a human being is egg-shaped. It extends approximately 90 cm (36 in) above the head, gradually diminishing in size until it closes under the soles of the feet. Inside this is a smaller cloak that extends about 10 cm (4 in) from the physical body and is known as the life-force field or etheric sheath (*see Figure 4.4 page 46*).

The Chakras

The human aura is comprised of many layers, each radiating its own ethereal colour. The etheric sheath is the layer nearest to the physical body and houses the energy channels (nadis), which absorb prana or life force from the atmosphere, and the energy centres or chakras.

There are seven main chakras situated at the border of the etheric body and known as lesser chakras. Each of these has its complementary chakra, known as the greater chakra, situated at the border of the aura. Very few of the people who have the gift of seeing auras can actually see the greater chakras.

The human chakras are, in an amazing way, made up of a complete rainbow. Basically, they are like the lenses of a telescope. Both the greater and the lesser chakras collect energy, or life force, from the aura. This is then conducted to the endocrine glands of the physical body. The chakras are like selective filters which select by way of colour. A single chakra never stands still. It follows a general pattern which can be strong and filled with life energy. It can also be temporarily weak. This usually shows in the brilliance or weakness of the colours. In Figure 4.1, 'A' indicates where the greater chakra is 'seen', or rather perceived, and 'B' how it passes through the lesser chakra.

Figure 4.1

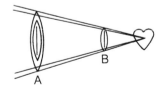

The Colour Order of the Chakras

The lesser chakras, situated in the etheric body, resemble a line of rotating discs which form a column of luminous light. Each one contains all the colours of the spectrum but displays one dominant colour. The first or base chakra displays red; the second or sacral chakra orange; the third or solar plexus chakra yellow; the fourth or heart chakra green; the fifth or throat chakra blue; the sixth or brow chakra indigo; and the seventh or crown chakra violet. Above these seven main chakras are three higher chakras which radiate magenta, white and the sacred darkness out of which all becomes manifest.

Knowing that each of the chakras, lesser and greater, contains all of the colours, let us take the heart chakra as an example to see how the colours are arranged.

It is the colour green that brings balance, cleansing, equilibrium and life renewal. Thus, the outermost layer of the heart chakra is green. In the order of the colour spectrum, the next colour layer will be turquoise, then blue, violet, magenta, red, orange and yellow at its centre (*see Figure 4.2*). This is the greater chakra order. The lesser chakra reverses this order showing yellow on the outside and green in the centre (*see Figure 4.3*). This system follows through each of the individual chakras in order to give life and vitality to each of the endocrine glands.

As the order of the colours of these two chakra systems is complementary, we can see that nature is responding to man's constant need for wholeness. Like a question and answer, this is the principle by which we find the instructions for our journey.

Figure 4.2

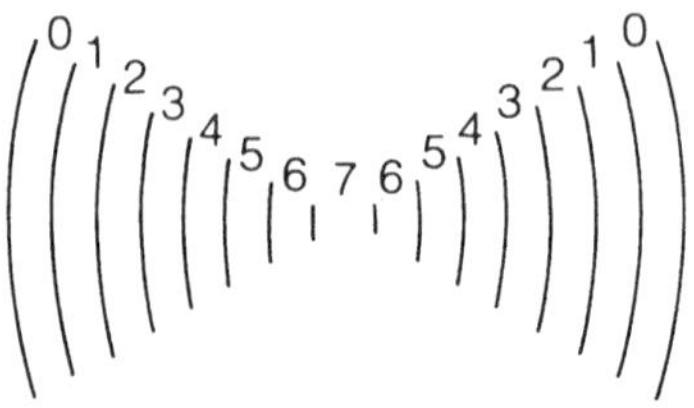

Figure 4.3

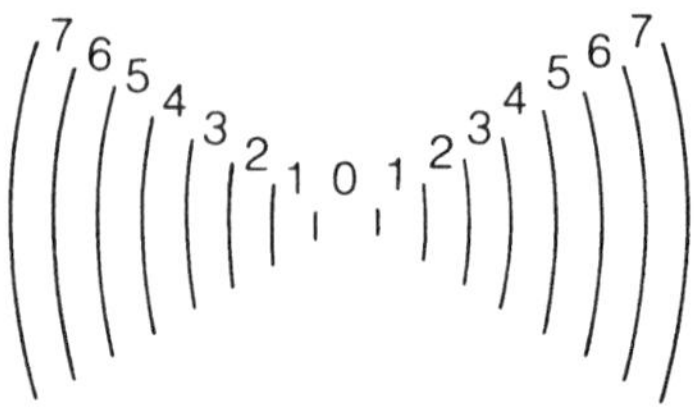

0 = the colour which represents the main colour of the aura, the remainder are as follows:

0 = the heart chakra = green

1 = yellow ☐   2 = orange   ☐ 3 = red ☐   4 = magenta ☐

5 = violet ☐   6 = blue   ☐ 7 = turquoise ☐

In this balance of the colours, we find in the middle of each chakra violet and magenta (*see Figure 4.2*). Violet denotes self-respect and dignity, and magenta denotes change and a letting go. These two colours work towards the spiritual energies which create the 'sacred heart', which gives a renewal rhythm to the bloodstream. The heart is usually understood to be the organ of love. The Christian Church connects the love of Jesus Christ to the heart and lifts this love into a more elevated love – without the slightest sexual implication – which is the Sacred Heart. This has no passion, only love for all living beings.

When we treat with colour, we take into account this renewal rhythm and use colour with its complementary. If this is not done, the body will respond negatively because the treatment is incomplete.

Practical Exercise

Take the other six chakras and work out their colour sequence. Discover the patterns associated with the greater and the lesser chakras. If you wish, you can then take a compass and draw eight ever-increasing circles on two separate sheets of paper and instead of putting numbers in the circles as illustrated in Figures 4.2 and 4.3, colour them with the appropriate colour. Replace 0 with 7 and 0 will then come into the place of 1. There will then be eight progressive pictures that will leave the spectrum intact but shift the colours so that red (base chakra) next time around becomes orange (adrenals), then yellow (solar plexus). This will give you drawings of all the chakras in turn and the outside colours will show that full-spectrum colour is the living colour of life.

In counselling, the most gentle suggestions are always far more acceptable than direct orders. Herbs and homoeopathic medicines are very successful because they also follow this principle of gentleness. By the same token, the more rarefied a colour, the better it works. By working with this principle, we offer the correct memory to the cell structure. The aura and the etheric sheaths surrounding minerals, plants, animals and humans are so fine that they still respond to thought patterns, emotions and general modes of movement. With good guidance from a professionally trained colour healer, we can learn how to conduct these forces to benefit health. The regular practice of certain colour visualizations is very successful in this respect. They rely precisely on immeasurably fine chemical and etheric changes which alter our often neglected behaviour patterns. Using colour visualization and coloured lights, the patient can learn to direct their own life force.

Aura Patterns

As well as radiating all the colours of the spectrum, the human aura contains energy patterns. These patterns change with diet, health, mood, emotional stability, etc. When a person is in good health, the chakras and energy patterns are in balance and the colours radiating in the aura are in harmony. In the following diagrams we start with the simple basic pattern of the aura.

Figure 4.4 shows the basic three areas with the physical body in the centre. The physical body has been able to manifest through the energies of the aura and the etheric sheath, both of which were present before the physical body came into being.

In all living things, there lies a beautiful principle behind all growth. Each year a tree puts around itself two rings of new life. One fast, short one in the summer and one slow, hard one in the winter. Likewise an onion comprises many skins. As illustrated in Figure 4.5, the 'invisible' structure of the aura comprises 'horizontal' layers. These layers or colours are called orbs and contain living shapes, for example the human body.

Where there are orbs or balls of energy, there is also a radiation pattern as indicated in Figure 4.6. Try to see this not in two-dimensional, but three-dimensional space.

Figure 4.4: The approximate size of the human aura:
A: Longest egg shape
B: Etheric sheath
C: The physical body

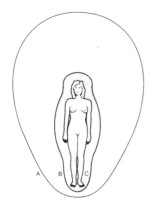

Figure 4.5: The aura with the horizontal layers.

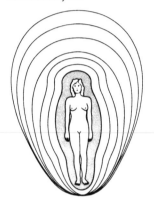

Figure 4.6: The aura with horizontal (orbs) and the vertical layers, or rays. These rays emanate energy from the chakra system.

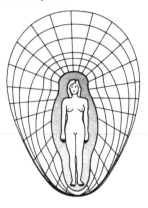

Figure 4.7: The aura showing the halo and wings.

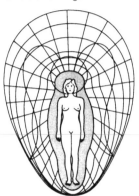

Potentially, we are all endowed with the most wonderful patterns. Everybody has a halo and wings in their aura. In some people these are quite pronounced, while in others they are only faint. More and more becomes visible to us if we ask questions, and when we are able to ask clear questions, the answers are forthcoming.

The number four is one of the most powerful numbers to anchor, to orientate and to secure mental, emotional, metabolic and physical structure, and the human body is no exception to this. Thus we have four main chakras built into the aura as in Figure 4.8. Two of these are acknowledged in the great gesture of blessing given by a priest when the palms of the hands are raised to bless the congregation. In the palms of the hands are also minor chakras and by allowing these to become channels of transmission, we are indeed using them to let the spiritual energies flow through.

In front of this wonderful 'cathedral' of our body (together with the aura, etheric sheath and all the beautiful structures within it) stands the bell tower, the church spire. In the case of the human person, this

Figure 4.8: The aura with wings and extra chakras, anchoring man into the four directions of space. These extra chakras, rather like the eyes on the wings of a peacock butterfly, support the whole of the auric energy.

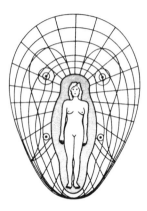

Figure 4.9: The aura with the column of chakras. In some teachings, taken from the Kabbalah, there are 18 chakras, but the ascending ninth chakra is overlapping here with the descending ninth chakra making a total of 17.

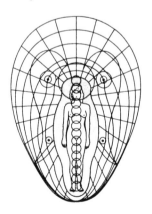

is the column of the chakras and it allows us to be conscious beings, standing upright, in proud humility, as my very dear teacher Father Andrew Glazewski would say.

Challenging Patterns

Frequently, distortions or discords can be found in the aura long before any physical disease appears. Signs that precede an illness can be detected there.

Before we refer to this as 'illness', we should remember that what we identify as a poison to the physical body can also be a remedy. In the ancient temples, alcohol and smoke were used to bring about certain states of mind. This was achieved via the metabolic system which, with the intake of alcohol, smoke or certain herbs, changes the personality.

In ancient times, the general pattern was not domination or politics, but a genuine, carefully conducted education or even initiation by the priests, who, incidentally, were also the doctors of the day. We are now living in a vastly matured and very sophisticated world where a great deal of mistrust has developed and where people have free access to drugs, cigarettes and alcohol.

Figure 4.10 shows how fine clouds of mist-type flecks develop when a person smokes cigarettes and drinks alcohol. An occasional cigarette or glass of wine or spirits can be cleared out of the aura within 24 hours. These cloudlike flecks lie horizontally and can be more easily removed by the vertical, radiating aura energy.

Figure 4.11 shows the aura 'pollution' that occurs through the use of hard drugs such as LSD or heroin. These drugs cause a type of damage to the aura that cannot be so easily eliminated. This is because the pollution is not a horizontally lying cloud, which is comparatively easy to disperse, but is like wedges or spears which cause cracks in the aura. Once these wedges have broken the aura there is no known remedy or cure.

We will now look at some of the patterns in the aura which are connected with the soul and mental aspect of a person. There are

Figure 4.10: The aura after smoking or drinking. It can be cleared after 24 hours unless the person is a chain smoker or an alcoholic.

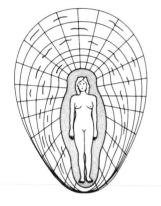

Figure 4.11: The aura showing the effect of hard drugs such as heroin.

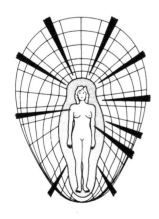

energies flowing in and out of the aura which we can and should accept because they are healing and revitalizing. When they are in harmony with the need of a person, they do not create a 'visible' mark in the aura. However, there are situations where on one level, even a subconscious level, a person does not accept the energies, thereby blocking their natural flow.

In Figure 4.12, instead of a fine, clear colour on each level of the aura we see what looks like a knotted ball of grey wool. This is blocking off the unaccepted energies. Grey is the colour of fear and untruth and can accumulate in the aura. However, it serves all the colours of the spectrum and creates space in which there is freedom to change. It can accept light (white) and darkness (black) and has a leaning towards silver.

When the opposite to Figure 4.12 happens, a person is unable to let negative energies which are no longer needed flow out of the aura. This also blocks up the aura (*see Figure 4.13*). It happens mainly to people who cannot give freely, who accrue wealth and hold on to possessions which they do not need. These people have a lot of brown in their aura. Brown is the colour of commitment. In the last resort it is the colour of death in the physical state. Brown has a leaning towards gold and is the colour that, in a way, dominates other colours. When living energy decays into the earth, it becomes dark brown humus. From this state new life can spring.

The conditions shown by Figures 4.12 and 4.13 respond very well to colour therapy from a qualified therapist. Counselling is also given, along with advice on how patients can help themselves.

There are many schools of thought on the aura and chakras and each one has a part to play. The basic principle is that there are energy patterns preceding any manifestation of living structures in all kingdoms of nature. As the human being becomes more and more aware, there appear more and more valuable insights, such as the number and the details of the chakras.

When I first started to perceive the aura, I saw just simple outlines and very little else. As I researched more deeply, more details

Figure 4.12: The aura showing the effect of energies not accepted by the thoughts, emotions or metabolic system. These gradually weaken the health structure and produce the colour grey, with the effect that the person often tends to opt out of life.

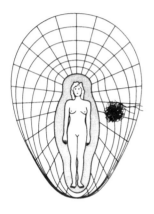

Figure 4.13: The aura showing the effect of energy not released from the body. If energy shows itself as brown, this indicates that it is no longer needed and should be discarded. If it stays in the aura, it will cause problems later.

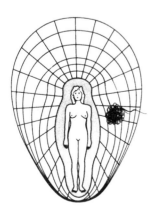

appeared. These always followed the original principle and laws of these phenomena. Figure 4.14 is based on two views that I have put together. The first is based on the teaching of the Kabbalah and the second is based on sacred geometry. The result of using both of these teachings is that we find a column of 18 chakras. Nine from the crown (the top of the head) down to the base chakra and nine rising from the soles of the feet to the base chakra, thus creating a wonderful mirror image which can be used for scanning (*see page 85*). The rising column covers the descending one at the base chakra, the sacred centre, where two human beings can become 'one flesh'. Those people who practise reflexology (zone therapy) will now see that the washing of feet by a master is not just an outward ceremony but that a healing action is being performed. (*See* John 13, v. 5, 'The washing of the feet by Christ'.)

A therapist who can perceive auras will sooner or later 'see' the image shown in Figure 4.15. This image shows how a stage of enlightenment can be found. There are no quick ways to learn how to perceive the aura or, for that matter, to become aware of the finer energy field around all manifested matter. Stones, plants, animals and humans all have an energy field; what needs to be learnt is how to make such 'vision' accessible. Through training, under the supervision and in the presence of a conscientious teacher, this 'double vibratory vision' can, however gradually, develop. Seeing the aura picture, either as a whole or in part, can happen suddenly, in which case a person quite unexpectedly finds themselves experiencing this vision capacity either momentarily or for longer periods. There are very fine means to help control such double vibratory vision: art therapy and good counselling. ECT, which causes it to 'shut down', should be avoided and only be used as a last resort, if at all. Personal dedication and very sound guidance are the only sure approaches to learning this double vibratory vision, and I must emphasize this.

Each of the seven chakras that are involved here is using the centre, the heart, to lift the more physical energies into the more

Figure 4.14: The scanning chart.

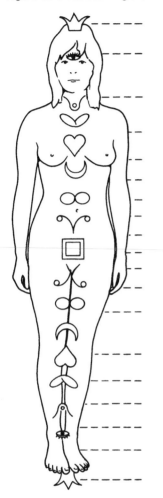

spiritual energies. Through this, a unification is achieved which brings us into contact with both the kingdom below us, the elemental world, and the kingdom above us, the angels (*see Chapter 7*). The colours which can be experienced range from very deep reds to very fine, almost invisible, magentas.

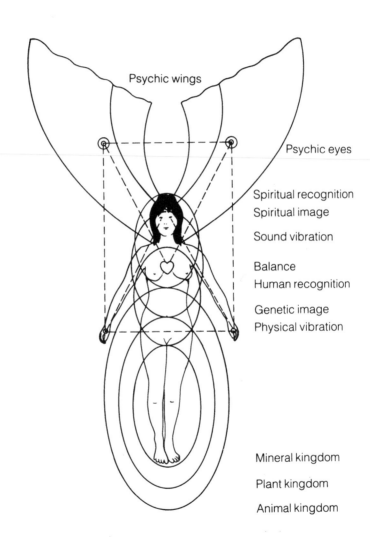

Psychic wings

Psychic eyes

Spiritual recognition
Spiritual image

Sound vibration

Balance
Human recognition

Genetic image
Physical vibration

Mineral kingdom

Plant kingdom

Animal kingdom

Figure 4.15: The raising of the centres, or chakras. It is possible to raise the chakras and enter a new dimension of energy so that the base chakra becomes the throat chakra, the sacral chakra the pituitary and the solar plexus chakra the crown. A conscientious, pure-hearted companion can raise you up into this higher vibration with one-to-one teaching.

The Two Complementary Rainbows

By now it should be clear to you that all things have their opposite or complementary image. Colour is no exception to this rule. Nature also reflects the innate phenomena of complementary energies. When we see a rainbow in the sky, there is always a complementary rainbow above it, although sometimes this is not visible to the human eye. The first rainbow mirrors and creates a second rainbow with the colours reversed (*see Figure 4.16*).

Through this we can personally experience that the spectrum is a circle of colour. The next time you see a rainbow, be very observant and look at the colours. If you see a second rainbow, take the trouble to compare the two. The first rainbow will have green at its centre and the second will have magenta at its centre. Here the magenta colour outshines the green that lies behind it. In the first rainbow, the green outshines the magenta. Because all of this is light, we cannot see through it. Also, coloured light cannot create colours such as grey and brown. These can only be created with pigment colours.

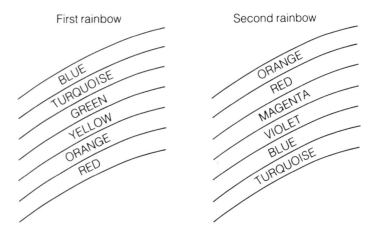

Figure 4.16: The two complementary rainbows.

Here we are entering an area which is the bridge or transition between the manifested solid world and the pre-manifested invisible world. Just as these beautiful colours can only appear for a comparatively short time, so all living energy is in the process of letting go of the past, moving into the present and on into the future. So, when we see the rainbow appear, we come from the past, into the present and we wonder at the phenomenon. It then disappears and is only left in our memory.

From the past, we can gather experiences which allow us to anticipate some future. When we gather the actual principles which stand behind all growth and all evolution, we can begin to see into the future. Variations and individual differences always signify that there is a law behind all living and loving events. When two energies meet at an equally measured strength and they are complementary, we can say that they create between them the third energy. It can be said that one and one make three and not two.

Take this same concept into music and we can start to hear that between an interval of two sounds lies the third energy. Sing an interval of a third or fifth twice. The first time sing it without a pause. The second time sing the same interval with a pause between the two notes. You will sense a tension. This tension we call energy. The longer the pause, the more you feel the energy. If you learn to listen between the various intervals contained in musical scales, you will notice that the energy changes with each interval. This energy between two sounds is actually the inaudible part of music, but, believe it or not, it is the healing part of the music.

The same principle applies with two colours when they are standing next to each other. They start to oscillate, creating an energy between them. Take eight pieces of different coloured paper (A4 size) and lay them next to each other without leaving a gap. Steadily look at them for up to 15 seconds. You will see that what is called a 'colour flash' arises. When the colours are 'neighbours', i.e. red and orange, green and turquoise, blue and violet, magenta and red or any

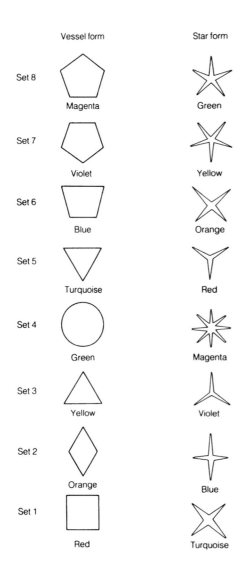

	Vessel form	Star form
Set 8	Magenta	Green
Set 7	Violet	Yellow
Set 6	Blue	Orange
Set 5	Turquoise	Red
Set 4	Green	Magenta
Set 3	Yellow	Violet
Set 2	Orange	Blue
Set 1	Red	Turquoise

Notes on complementary energy

Human consciousness arises out of the swing between extremes, light–dark, hot–cold, etc. This polarity principle is built into all things which we encounter. Thus, the vessel form (the feminine) has also the star form (the masculine) within. Neither has a purpose unless they actually relate to each other. Complementary forms are supported by complementary colours and sound is no exception. Both sound and the listening have to co-operate, sound being the masculine aspect and the listening being the feminine. Explore further and find yourself standing right between these forces of polarity, constantly struggling to keep the balance. The vessel containers should fit in to each other perfectly: if the vessel is too small the content breaks it, if it is too large then the content is lost in it.

Figure 4.17: Vessel form and star form
The energy of form is again a double energy and goes back to the ancient (sacred) geometry known to master builders. The vessel form (container) is linked to feminine energy, and the complementary star form is aligned to male energy. The syllable 'gon' denotes the vessel and 'gram' the star, such as hexagon and hexagram (*see* Critchlow, 1969). These terms come from the Greek. Each aperture changes the grid of light and thereby conducts the colour in a new way each time. Basically all 'window' are apertures and, according to their shape, change the light grid and create a certain atmosphere inside a room. (*See also* 'The colour consciousness set', *page 81*.)

of the mixtures which are possible between the eight colours, the energies are gentle. When, however, you use orange and violet or red and green, turquoise and yellow, you find certain discords. The possible third order is to use complementary colours only, such as red and turquoise, orange and blue, yellow and violet, etc. With these there appears a wonderful complementary energy that seems to satisfy the sense of sight and brings about harmony, not tension. Work with these eight colours and find out which combination is most enjoyable for you.

Now look at the instructions on the energies of each colour (*see pages 21–3*). You may learn something about yourself. It is most likely that at this moment in time you need the colours which you have chosen in order to satisfy a need within yourself. Say, for instance, that you have chosen a violet and a blue. Look at the meanings and apply them to yourself. Are you currently in need of self-respect and dignity? Has someone or something taken this valuable energy away from you? Do you also require peace and relaxation? Have you not allowed time for yourself but have been running around in circles? Allow these colours to be visualized within you.

Try to work out whether this requirement is momentary, temporary or for a longer duration. You may come to feel that you need violet and yellow to create a balance within yourself, or, alternatively, blue and orange.

Blue and orange are two very special colours. They appear when you have achieved peace (blue) and joy (orange) in yourself. If this applies through your whole being, body, mind and spirit, then you have achieved a wonderful harmony. Through experience, these colours have been found to be linked with children under eight years of age and in adults who are natural healers. Just imagine you are filled with peace, relaxation, joy and happiness. What else do you need? A relaxed, joyful person, free from tension, becomes a pure instrument for healing energies to flow through them.

Chapter 5

Rhythms in Colour

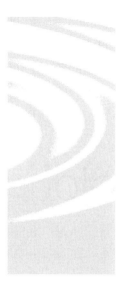

MEPHISTOPHELES: Since thou O Lord again approaches
Asking how all is shaping up down here
And thou art by and large well pleased to see me.
Thus I am also part of this assembly ...

J. M. Goethe, Prologue in Heaven, Faust 1

All life, including human beings and our planet, needs a challenge. This is the reason why we need the complementary energies which are inherent in all living beings.

Life depends upon the very fine balance of the colours and their complementary colours. It is when the balance of health is upset that colour therapy is given to restore harmony in the body. This is made possible because our biochemical structure is light-sensitive.

The very first colour-therapy instrument I made was programmed to administer two minutes of the necessary colour interlaced with two minutes of its complementary colour (five on the increasing scale, four on the decreasing scale). This made nine changes, each change being of two minutes' duration. However, when I discovered this was not working I used a skin galvanizer and a blood pressure gauge that gave no response after the third change on the colour-therapy instrument. This showed that the human body reacts very quickly to mechanical rhythms and 'switches off' when there is no more to be learnt.

The Fibonacci Series of Proportions

While I was designing what came to be known as our colour space illuminator, I was thinking about proportions. These should always be observed in design and I based the design of this lamp on the proportions of the Golden Mean. These rhythmic proportions were discovered by Fibonacci (qv), an eleventh-century monk who lived in Pisa, Italy. His original series of numbers were:

$$1 + 1 = 2$$
$$1 + 2 = 3$$
$$2 + 3 = 5$$
$$3 + 5 = 8$$
$$5 + 8 = 13$$
$$8 + 13 = 21$$
$$13 + 21 = 34 \text{ etc.}$$

Figure 5.1: The common stinging nettle. This displays very clearly the Golden Mean proportions, the rhythms in space which we now use for time.

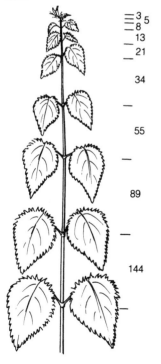

These proportions are found in crystals, plants, animals and humans (*see Figure 5.1*). I felt that integrating them into the design of the colour space illuminator made it into something very special.

Suddenly I realized that time and space are interchangeable. So why not transfer the Golden Mean proportions into time for use with the colour-therapy instrument? I worked with this idea and came up with a time-change sequence that was aligned to the vibrational harmony of the human body. I also realized that this sequence is deeply embedded in all nature. The sequence is as follows.

The instrument begins with a short 45-second exposure of the therapy colour and is followed with a $3^{1}/_{4}$ minute exposure of the complementary colour. With each change, the therapy colour

Figure 5.2: The colour space illuminator.

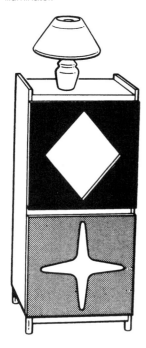

increases from 45 seconds to 1¹/4 minutes, 2 minutes, 3¹/4 minutes, ending with a 5¹/4 minute exposure.

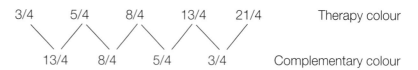

This totals 12¹/2 minutes. In between each of these five exposures, the complementary colour appears in a diminishing order. It goes from 3¹/4 minutes down to 2 minutes to 1¹/4 minutes and ends with ³/4 minute. This totals 7¹/4 minutes, making the complete treatment time 19³/4 minutes.

$12.5 \div 7.25 = 1.724$.

The rhythm produced by these time changes is a total Golden Mean rhythm. It presents a surprise element to the body which motivates the cell structure to expand and contract. Because all of the changes have a different time interval, the rhythm becomes alive and not mathematical.

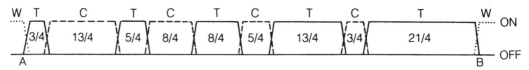

Figure 5.3: Graph of the rhythms of the instrument.

Explanation and key
The indicated fractions are ¹/4 of a minute. The following letters are:
W – Working light switched on manually.
A – Start of treatment operated by the therapist.
T – Treatment colour time on the increase.
C – Complementary colour time on the decrease.
The crossing over indicates fade-in and fade-out (2 secs).

At the end of the treatment (19³/4 mins) the working light will come on automatically to signify the actual finish of the treatment. We have indicated to the patient before the therapy has started that there is no rush to get up after the treatment has ended.

How to Make a Chart to Determine the Colour for Therapy

The central energy on which all things are based manifests in orbital form and in linear rays of light issuing from the centre to the periphery three-dimensionally. In crystal growth it is multi-dimensional but in a geode it frequently streams from the periphery to the centre. In plants it is more orientated towards a vertical direction. In animals it is horizontal (based on the position of the spine). In humans during wakefulness and daily work it is vertical and during sleep, like the animals, horizontal. The spine is our central column of energy, which is linked to the brain. Each vertebra has an outlet to the organs in the chest and trunk of the body, and also to the arms and legs. The spinal cord supplies the body with sensitivity and the necessary functions for our daily life.

The human capacity for communication is extremely complex. It can take place by looking at another person, by shaking hands, kissing or embracing. If the last two are deepened it can, at the right time and for the right purpose for the particular individuals, lead to the holy act of love making.

A person's vibration is contained in their handwriting, a lock of their hair, a drop of their blood or a photograph of them. In times past and even today, a couple may exchange a lock of hair in order to be in touch with each other. If you travel away from home and are inclined to become homesick, it can help if you carry in a pouch a small piece of earth from your own garden. When you write a letter by hand, you put part of yourself into it and this remains for a long time. When some of the natives of Africa or America, for example, refuse to be photographed, it is because they have a deep inner feeling that something is being taken away from them. In a sense this is correct, but if we have their consent, then it is permissible.

The ancient art of using these very fine energies to heal or to communicate is known as dowsing. With this art we can establish a communication between ourselves and our patient. This can give us very accurate information about a patient, provided that we are able to exercise complete detachment from the patient. Because of this need for detachment, it is very difficult to dowse for someone who is very close to us, such as wife or husband, mother and very close friends, people whom we regularly care for or work with where a bond exists, either emotionally or physically.

Dowsing for Colour Therapy

When one thinks about dowsing, the picture that comes to mind is of a person holding a rod or forked stick (as in *Figure 5.4*). This is held loosely in both hands. The person then walks over the area where they have been asked to locate water, minerals, oil or metals. When a source has been located, the rod will move upward or downward.

The dowser can then determine the quality and amount of the substance by asking questions. A clear question will always receive the response 'yes' or 'no'; when the formulation of a question is not clear, bewilderment – 'I don't know' – follows. So you have to say, for example: 'Is there a spring in this field?' If the answer is no, you will have to go to the next field. If yes, the next question is: 'Is it straight ahead towards the opposite gate?' If yes, walk on and at one point the rod will react. The next question becomes: 'How deep is the spring? 'Is it 10 ft?' No reaction. 'Is it 17 ft?' Yes. The reaction is telling us that at 17 ft there is a spring. Next questions: 'How much water per hour?' '60 gall?' '40 gall?' 'Is it pure?' 'Is it lasting?' etc. In this way a very clear, detailed and precise picture can be built up.

Dowsers are used more widely than is generally known. Their skills can save many industries a lot of money. It is even possible to locate lost property by this method.

Dowsing can also be used to locate problems in a human being. In colour therapy, we dowse to find the precise colours that are needed to harmonize a person's health.

Figure 5.4: Dowsing.

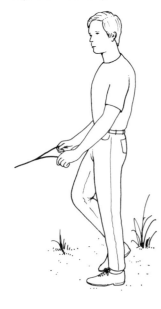

The Hygeia Spine Chart

We are ourselves fields of energy in which the spine is the central source. If we take the human spine and include the eight flat bones of the skull, which can be looked upon as metamorphosed vertebrae, this gives us a total of 40 vertebrae. But, these eight flat bones of the skull are not used in colour therapy.

The remaining 32 are used and these are divided equally into four major areas, each area represented by eight vertebrae. The seven cervical and first thoracic represent the mental aspect of a person. The next eight thoracic represent the emotional area. The remaining three thoracic and the five lumbar represent the metabolic area, and the sacrum, which before it became fused contained eight vertebrae, represents the physical body. Each of these four sections contains the eight colours of the spectrum, one colour for each vertebra. The colours in the mental area are very light, but as we come down the spine they gradually become darker, ending with very strong colours in the sacrum.

If we, as therapists, are dowsing for a fellow human being in order to try and help them, the first thing we have to do is to raise our level of consciousness to the state where we are able to become detached from our personal and daily problems.

One of the ways of doing this is to confirm within ourselves what our intentions are and then to light a white candle on behalf of the work that we are about to undertake. We then take a chart of the human spine (*Figure 5.5*) and ask the patient to sign it on the back, along the spine. Their signature acts as a 'witness' because it contains their energy and it is this that we are able to pick up. We then dowse out each individual vertebra. To do this, the middle finger of the non-dominant hand is used. Most people are right-handed so they use the left hand. Raising the arm away from the chest, we allow the middle finger to hover about half an inch above the diagram of the spine, making sure that the finger does not come into contact with the paper. Where a reaction is felt in the finger – and this can take the

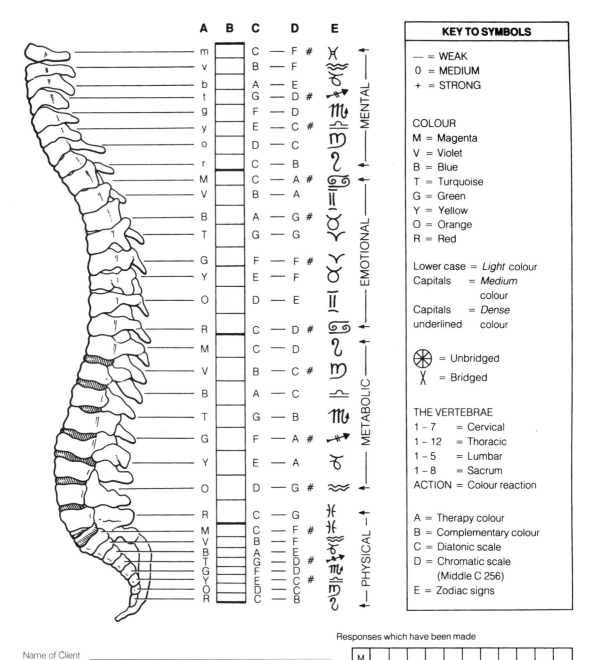

KEY TO SYMBOLS

— = WEAK
0 = MEDIUM
+ = STRONG

COLOUR
M = Magenta
V = Violet
B = Blue
T = Turquoise
G = Green
Y = Yellow
O = Orange
R = Red

Lower case = *Light* colour
Capitals = *Medium* colour
Capitals underlined = *Dense* colour

⊕ = Unbridged
Ⴟ = Bridged

THE VERTEBRAE
1 – 7 = Cervical
1 – 12 = Thoracic
1 – 5 = Lumbar
1 – 8 = Sacrum
ACTION = Colour reaction

A = Therapy colour
B = Complementary colour
C = Diatonic scale
D = Chromatic scale
(Middle C 256)
E = Zodiac signs

Responses which have been made

M									
E									
ME									
PH									

Name of Client _____

Date of Chart _____ Made by _____ (Signed)

Time _____ Treatment Colour _____

Weather _____

Figure 5.5: The medical colour diagnosis chart.

M – mental; ME – metabolic; E – emotional; PH – physical

form of pain, heat, cold or a prickling sensation – the relevant vertebra on the spine chart is marked with a cross in the centre.

Colour Counselling

In very advanced scientific circles it is known that the thoughts and emotions of a scientist control the end result of their work. The more refined the structures they use, the more likely it is that the outcome will be very different each time the experiment is conducted. This shows that each person has individual harmony patterns which are not acceptable to anyone else.

Colour therapy is based on many of these ideas and can often prove them. When we learn to visualize, to sense the effects of colour, learn to think colour, then we can create certain experiences. When there is conflict between people and one of them visualizes a deep strong blue into this conflict, it is quite often surprising how quickly the conflict dissolves. Conflict comes out of misunderstanding. When we are challenged on this we become insecure and try to defend ourselves. This causes tension which in turn causes contraction within the body. The colour associated with contraction is red. Blue is the colour of expansion and relaxation and this is the reason why this colour causes the conflict to dissolve.

If a person is aware of tension in a fellow human being, they can restore peace and calm in them by visualizing the colour of blue and projecting it out in the pattern of a figure of eight to the person in need of help (see Figure 5.6).

As A sends the energy of blue through B, all of B's negative energy is anchored and the uplifting effect that the blue energy contains brings calm and ease to B. This can only be done successfully if A exercises detachment and is working purely for the good of B and not for their own self-esteem. What is projected from B is acknowledged and anchored on the low point of the figure of eight. This

Figure 5.6: Projecting colour in the pattern of a figure of eight. The person who transmits the healing is first drawing in from the higher self the energies which are then offered to the person who needs this help. Through this action the 'patient' is related back to their own higher self and finds that a refreshing healing occurs.

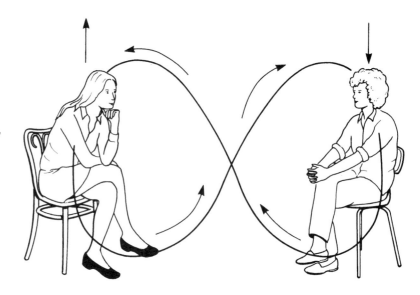

ensures that no negativity is returned to A. This is a technique of silent communication and, according to the energies wished for, can also be used with other colours. All those who have done this will know how successful it is.

I was once a member of a training group run by a leader who challenged each of us to express the way in which we worked with people. A chaplain complained that he didn't get very much response from the people he interviewed. The leader asked him to explain how he started his interviews. The chaplain said that when the person sat in front of him, into his mind would come thoughts such as: 'This is "Aunty", "Charlie", "The Joker", "Misery Guts" etc.'

The leader then challenged the chaplain to give each of the 16 people in the group a title. The chaplain was delighted by this and had successfully gone halfway round the circle when he came to me. He looked at me and said, 'Oh, this is Aladdin and I trust him not.'

He then moved on to the young woman who was next to me and said, 'She is "benevolent" mum.'

At this point he broke down in tears and could not continue. The leader allowed a little time for him to regain his composure. During this time, from where I was sitting, I made a figure of eight, sending calm and relaxation to him. Obviously, no one knew what I was doing. The leader then asked the chaplain to choose two people from the group whom he would like to counsel him and help him to find a new technique for his interviews. The chaplain chose 'benevolent mum' and me, whom he had previously said he did not trust.

Many more such cases could be quoted. But what one has to remember is that this technique must never be used for self-advantage.

It cannot be said often enough that the moment you use any therapy, you become the channel for the energy of that therapy to flow from your higher self through you. When you apply this to a fellow human being, you are under a very strict obligation to observe all your own thoughts, feelings and actions (again, a three-fold principle). All the training and all the learning, together with the practical work which was done during your study, have become your expertise. Like a good pianist, you no longer have to think how to apply your method of healing on a practical level. The use of your fingers, arms, instruments, lamps or coloured sheets are in your cell memory. This part of your work has become automatic, leaving space in your thoughts to interpret what is happening between you and your patient.

I use the word 'interpret' because you are no longer using your intellect, you are using your intuition to sense the interplay between you and your patient. The colours which you apply are active energies. They are working to bring a harmonious balance to the patient. However, every single application, every hour, day, time and meeting is a new experience and the events which they bring are unique. You may repeat what you have done so many times before but each treatment can, and indeed does, unlock new doors for both patient and therapist.

The therapist is the specialist who has to interpret what is now happening. So observe, listen, sense, perceive, as if you were watching a play in the theatre. Make notes of what you feel is happening and, at the appropriate moment, tell the patient.

During a treatment a patient can enter into a new stage of their being. At the correct time, a point will be reached when all circumstances meet together.

The time is right.
The patient is ready to open up to the treatment.
The therapist becomes a perfect channel.
Suddenly something happens which the patient and the therapist
    have 'waited for'.

Such moments are very special and miracles can happen. At such a moment, the following dedication, which the therapist can use, has been fully realized.

'I am in the right place
At the right time
For the right purpose.'

Chapter 6

The Healing Light

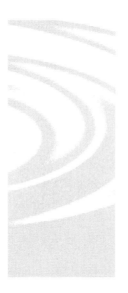

... and the light shone into darkness and the darkness comprehended it not ...

John 1, v. 1

We have in the preceding chapters explored light and colours and talked about darkness. And there has been an underlying assumption that light and colour are all registered through the eyes. But the sense of sight is only one part of our seeing capacity; our eyes are only part of this sense. All our cells are light-sensitive and the human body is transparent; the pigments of our skin, our organs and even our bones are not insensitive to the changes of day and night, although we have to measure this using degrees of opaqueness.

Practical Exercise

If you can, go into a small room where there is only one small window. Close the door and put a black piece of paper over the window so that it is absolutely dark. Cut a hole in the paper no bigger than the palm of your hand. On a bright sunny day, cover this hole with your hand and very soon you will find that a very small orange light is created as you look at the patch that you have covered. This is actually the complementary colour to the daylight blue of early afternoon.

The most healing light is daylight because it contains the full spectrum – all the visible range of light is part of the illumination. It holds all the colours in it, but because it is so bright it is often said to be white light.

Practical Exercise

Shine a red light onto a white screen or wall. Add a blue light partly overlapping the red light. Now add a green light partly overlapping the first two. At the point where all three overlap, you will not get a mixture of the three colours but a white light *(see Figure 6.1)*.

Each coloured light that is added to the existing lights will make the area lighter and in the end create white light, although only red, blue and green filters are used. For this you will need the following: three torches, one of each of the following colour filters (which Hygeia can supply; these are of high quality and are not cheap): blue, red, green; you may also add orange, yellow, violet, etc.; a white screen some 60 cm x 60 cm (24 in x 24 in) and washing pegs. Black out your room and see how your colours are mixing.

If you repeat this using paint or crayons, the place where all three colours overlap will now become a very dark area, and not white as experienced with light *(see Figure 6.2)*. Each pigment adds further darkness to the existing pigments. This only becomes clear when you work with watercolours, which are transparent.

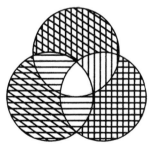

Figure 6.1: The subtractive colours.

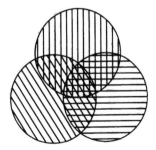

Figure 6.2: The additive colours.

The colour of light has a very special effect when we take into consideration its complementary colour, which always appears in its own shadow. For example, if a yellow light is shone onto a tree, the shadow produced by that tree would appear as violet. The purity of the light shone on the tree ascertains the purity of its shadow colour. Coloured shadows can be very deceptive, but also very beautiful.

Absolute light and absolute shadow do not exist since these concepts are always relative. However, where light and shadow, day and night meet in morning and evening – we can experience colours. The blue end of the spectrum appears in the morning and the red end during sunset. Man can extract from nature that which he deems useful to his ends. Whether this is beneficial or detrimental depends very much on the motives and purpose behind any development.

Artificial Light

Artificial light started with fire to illuminate the darkness, followed by the candle and the torch, all of which caused a high incidence of red, thereby distorting the daylight colours (daylight is actually blue). When we use artificial light, we should aim to get as near as possible to daylight, the living light that offers us a wonderful life-enhancing environment.

When Edison invented the household tungsten lamp, he left us with a standard colour of illumination for many decades. This contained a high red content. Much changed with the advent of fluorescent light. This gave us a very bright light at a much reduced energy cost since the greater part of the electric current is converted into light and not heat.

Society has a great need for economy and fluorescent light sources provide this admirably. However, artificial light which has been developed for economical reasons does not take into consideration its effect upon the mental, emotional and even physical well-being of the people who are subjected to it.

I knew the scientist Dr Hans Heitler, who developed fluorescent light in the early 1930s. He pronounced that it was not a healthy light, labelling it as emergency illumination only, 'economy light' that 'must not be used in peacetime'.

This warning has not been adhered to and we have subjected a whole generation to a light source that can cause stress, whether it be in the office, or in public places such as shops and stores, or from street lighting.

The reason why fluorescent light causes stress is because it is based on a gas filament and not on an alloy glowing one. The AC (alternating current) has a cycle of 50 to 50 on/off vibration. The human eye cannot see this fast flicker. However, the nerve ends of the skin pick it up subconsciously, which causes the brain and nervous system to vibrate in a mechanical rhythm. It causes headaches, deterioration of eyesight and general stress. Dr John Ott took Heitler's work and found that an improvement is possible when the hue and the very basic production method are carefully considered. From this, he developed a full-spectrum tube that has no colour distortions.

During the 1970s and early 1980s we developed, with the help of a very good international firm, a component now known as the electronic ballast, which has removed the unhealthy 'flicker' from the fluorescent tube. In this way, we are no longer subjected to the detrimental 50 Hz flicker of ordinary fluorescent lights.

It is thanks to Dr John Ott that we have the full-spectrum fluorescent tubes available today. All of these, with the exception of 8 ft tubes, can be operated by electronic ballast. Daylight is endowed with full-spectrum frequency and electronically ballasted full-spectrum tubes produce near-perfect light for all biochemical structures, plants, animals and humans. The cheaper, poor illumination which we generally install may well have to be paid for later in repairing the damage to health.

Public Lighting

We know that light and behaviour patterns are very closely linked. My company has been concerned with colour and its effect on living structure since 1956, when, as its founder, I first investigated colours and their use for human health in a small cellar near Bristol. Since diiferent colours vibrate at different frequencies, the effect of colours on people also varies and can be positive or negative in character. The red end of the spectrum has a frequency of about 4.6×10^{14} and, as already mentioned, causes contraction in all biochemical structures. The blue end, with a frequency of about 7.5×10^{14}, causes expansion. Red, in other words, causes excitement, stress, high blood pressure and tension. All green objects become black under red illumination and all red objects become white.

The effect of light and colour on behaviour patterns is of particular relevance with regard to public lighting. Low-pressure sodium light turns most colours into dirty greys and khaki. Thus the night scene in a city street with this monochromatic sodium light is a very negative environment for the inhabitants. The shadows of this light are a dirty maroon–grey. Violet, its beautiful clear neighbour in the spectrum, is the colour of dignity and respect, and when this is distorted into the unclean colour of a muddy maroon–grey it evokes psychological responses that cause people without positive motivations or plans to adopt an attitude of violent destructive craving. Similarly, while sexuality can be the highest form of human dignified expression, in such an environment it can become the lowest and most desecrated activity. Records show that in areas where education has failed to create a worthwhile daily life, 'floundering' people are easily provoked into destroying positive activities and objects which are, to them, a challenge they cannot live up to. Sex crimes of the most unpleasant kind can be the result of this.

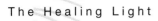

So, street lighting can cause depression in disoriented humans who quite frequently are under the influence of drink, smoking and drugs. This kind of lighting creates in their emotions and subconscious a tendency to 'drag down' all that is still positive in them. They are often not alone in their suffering, having others whom they have forced into this negative state. Gang leaders need weak followers whom they can bully.

There is no justification in describing the above phenomenon unless we can come up with a helping hand to improve matters. Improvements may require investment and a willingness to take a long-term view. They may not immediately pay off and should not, therefore, be considered as an emergency measure. However, if we invest now we will see a better future where fewer offences are committed and the police are better supported. Any increase towards better colour rendition and full-spectrum illumination would be helpful, but a street light in which the spectrum of light is more towards the blue end would be ideal. Blue is the colour of relaxation and peace; blood pressure is lowered and slow movement is induced, stress is removed and violence greatly reduced. In 1974 I made two suggestions to the police: that they should create blue-lit exit tunnels from football grounds through which all spectators would have to pass on leaving or that there should be a secondary illuminationcircuit which would flood the ground with blue light towards the end of the match. As far as I know, neither suggestion has been taken up and the violence and hysteria at some matches have led to the loss of life.

Colour and Effect

Any light, including public lighting, always manipulates a response. If it is well designed and based on deeper understanding, it will influence people towards better behaviour. Basically, light creates new ambiences and is able to change an environment, just as theatrical lighting changes the mood on stage. Artificial illumination creates vast pockets of shadow; shadow areas challenge the mind and emotions. The colour of such shadows invites certain activities which one could say are lured out of emotions and become urges. Undirected people are finally provoked into turning these urges into action. It would be quite a study to examine all night crimes in terms of the light and shadow present at the scene of each crime.

Very fine degrees of a mixture of shades can change the meanings of colour to an individual. These meanings cannot be put into concepts, far less into words.

The complexity of each individual psyche ensures a very personal appraisal of colour and therefore it is not easy to make generalizations beyond what has been outlined above. However, through the many years of my research I can say that on the whole the following effects can be experienced. Colours impress children very strongly, both boys and girls, as they are very pliable. A colour experienced at a very happy moment can remain a favourite for decades. Conversely, a bad moment associated with colour in early years can remain negative for an equally long time. The conscious acceptance of a bad experience can solve negative attitudes, however, and a 'bad' colour can become agreeable. Any experience, whether mental or emotional, can introduce itself into our health pattern and become a physical change, thereby altering our well-being. This can lead to disease as well as to health.

It has become fashionable recently to experiment with different colours in both the decoration and illumination of rooms. However, colour manipulation which is applied through the intellect without taking into account the philosophy of the colour principles will not work. The prison cell painted pink, for example, which is said to calm violent behaviour, has a very extreme backlash. The biochemical structure is forced into an extreme order to which it is not normally subjected. Pink is nearest to magenta, the first colour that emerges out of ultraviolet. It promotes change, letting go, dissolving, giving up.

Out of these qualities comes the relaxing of violent behaviour. Afterwards, however, there is a backlash of intense rebellion and violence. So what have we achieved? The pink cell is not actually a colour treatment, it is an emergency action, and, like a bad chess player, we have not taken into account the ensuing moves of our opponent.

Man has a double nature: one is rational, logical, orderly and creates reason; the other is intuitive, artisitic, playful and cannot be contained in strictly reasonable terms. We also have to take into account our nervous system: the brain has two halves, one mathematical (left side) and the other intuitive and artistic (right side). In our present educational system, far too much emphasis is still placed on the mathematical and logical side. We neglect the intuitive, which contains all the arts, music, painting, drama, etc. Many young people miss out at school as they are not mentally suited to academic work. They become failures and end up with no place in society. As they become vulnerable to all the influences of the environment, they become increasingly at odds with a society they have failed to please and often turn to crime, especially in the deprived city areas. But ultimately, through this behaviour to society, they are saying, 'I am also here. Acknowledge me.'

The colour of light plays a vital part in improving behaviour. The perfect colour would be daylight equivalent full-spectrum, in other words blue light such as in daylight tubes. The incandescent lamp has one great advantage: it neither goes fully out nor fully on. The effect is a cycle between on and off that does not touch the extreme on either side (*see Figure 6.3*).

Reams have been written, arguments have been proved and contradicted over the use of light in industry, commerce and entertainment. Yet deep-down there is a feeling of what is right and wrong. This has been built into and passed on to our cell structure for millennia. This cell memory tells us that light is vibrating at a constant frequency, at such a high frequency of the electromagnetic spectrum

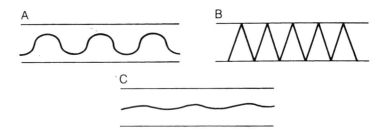

Figure 6.3: Incandescent, fluorescent and 'perfect' light patterns. 'A' is the incandescent lamp. 'B' is the unprotected, not electronically ballasted, fluorescent lamp or tube. 'C' is the 'perfect' light which we can now have.

that it goes into quintillions of vibrations per second. The finest of all human sensitivity can only recognize it as a calming, steady light that burns without interruption.

Any rhythm we put into this has an effect upon us. Therefore, we must find out what should be the correct rhythm. Nothing can be perfect, but we do now have at our disposal the means to achieve much better lighting conditions. We could ensure that stress through lighting is at a minimum and that work and leisure can be experienced by way of colour at a calm and peaceful level. This will, in turn, improve work output, quality of work, and the elimination of errors which can occur within seconds and take hours to correct.

The colour of light slips very quickly into the subconscious cell memory, whereas the colour in decoration stays with us mentally. These two can, and must, be used in conjunction with each other if interior design is to be successful. Since we have within us the complementary reactions of our brain functions, and since we are on this planet as men and women (i.e. two complementary energies), this principle of duality must be adopted so as to harmonize the environment and through it improve human communication. Very high illumination levels bring about non-communication among groups of people. So we should use light in a very subtle way, with a very carefully chosen colour and the well-considered decoration of living and working space.

Much research still has to be done before we can come up with a constructive design. Balance has always to be maintained, for harmonious intercommunication can emerge from it for the purpose of

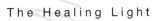

increasing life's benefits and for the sake of real lighting development which will benefit all concerned. Professionals who are in charge of illumination should increase their understanding of what good colour lighting can achieve.

Ways of Using Colour

Most people take light and illumination for granted and do not realize the major contribution it makes to physical and emotional well-being. We all have natural rhythms which are aligned to the natural environment. Basically, we require daylight to stimulate our senses (activity) and a natural darkness to give relaxation (sleep). People who work in a highly lit environment should also spend a lot of time in darkness.

In the technological world of today, we are being forcibly divorced from our natural rhythms. Broadly speaking, agricultural workers are the only people whose work allows them to remain aligned to their environment. Millions of people working in offices and factories can only feel the influences of natural light at short, odd intervals during the day. A considerable number of people on night work, or who work underground, are not afforded even the odd interval. Such a divorce considerably undermines our chance of well-being. It is further undermined through our being subjected to artificial lighting which, almost invariably, has been installed by people who do not know about its adverse physical or emotional effects.

When we become aware that colour and light can help us to be more harmonious and support our health, then we can ask how these can be employed to help us.

The Water Solarizer

An old and very well-known way to bring colour into the body is one practised in Ayurvedic medicine.

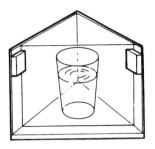

Figure 6.4: The water solarizer.

Very simply, encase a glass of spring water all round with quality full-spectrum glass made with pure oxides (you can order this from Lamberts in Germany – *see Resources*). Expose this to daylight for an hour when the sun is shining or two to three hours on a cloudy day (*see Figure 6.4*). By doing this you will change the chemical make-up of the water. Red glass will cause the water to taste slightly sour and blue glass will make the same quality of water taste sweetish. The red-treated water has an energizing effect if taken regularly, say, a few sips every ten minutes. It will make you feel more active. The blue water will relax you. In this way you can begin to help yourself.

You can use any of the colours of the rainbow to solarize your spring water. To help with arthritic conditions, use yellow glass, use green for cleansing, turquoise to strengthen your immune system, etc. Refer to Chapter 3 to find the colour needed for a specific complaint (*see pages 21–3*). These methods are gentle, however, and will cause a gradual alteration and not an abrupt one. Do not lose patience when working with this method. Your 'problem' has come gradually and gradually it will go away.

The Colour Consciousness Set

Colours cause responses within us and the eye strengthening chart shown in Chapter 3 can be extended to include all the rainbow colours. This is done with the aid of the 'colour consciousness' set (*see Figure 6.5*). This set contains 24 plates which, when worked with, improve the entire nervous system and help your memory. They are also good for impaired eyesight and help counteract the after effects of stroke, loss of speech and paralysis. The set contains very special geometric shapes, linking it to mathematics and thereby appealing to the brain functions. Our left-brain orientated Western education causes people to learn to judge and calculate, often to their own advantage, regardless of the environment as a whole, not to mention fellow humans. Beauty and art, colours and their energies

Figure 6.5: The colour consciousness set. These eight shapes and complementary shapes are made up into three sheets of each of the eight colours. The colour is always recognized with the right brain (the imaginative side of our brain), whereas the shape or geometric forms are registered on the left side of the brain (the logical side). These 24 colour prints are collated into Colour Consciousness Sets (*see Resources*).

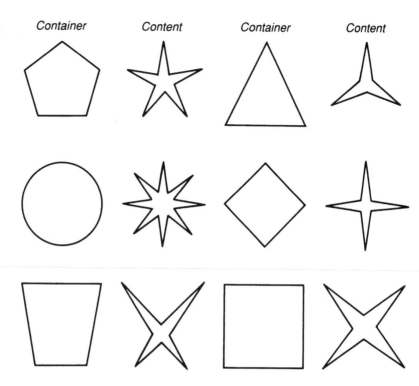

Container   *Content*   *Container*   *Content*

appeal to the right side of the brain, the intuitive, imaginative energies within us. By putting together colour and form (shapes) in a meaningful sequence we can create harmony and enliven our own being.

Colours, as you now know, are linked to their complementary colours. This phenomenon is not only restricted to colour but reappears also in form. When working with the colour consciousness set, you are continuously activating both the left and the right side of the brain.

The complementary colour range should by now be well known to you. The same principle is experienced when we examine forms. Forms have complementary forms by way of their tension energy. Each edge of a form has a given tension but the most powerful tension is the diagonal, to start with not seen but experienced.

Your brain is not a heap of cells of which you use only one tenth, as it is said, but a very fine organ that responds to your consciousness level and you can be in charge of it. Crossing from one side of the brain to the other will bring more life into your thought capacity, enabling you to gradually improve your creativity.

The Hygeia Pure Light Lamp

Our sense of sight has to cope with many negative aspects in this day and age and so light should be of good quality. Hygeia Studios has developed a good reading and working lamp which is known as the Hygeia pure light lamp (*see Figure 6.6*).

This lamp is an important source of illumination for artists, printers, dressmakers and for all those who are concerned with colour. The light is far less tiring on the eyes than the usual light.

Eyestrain often occurs when one is constantly under illumination that contains a high incidence of the red spectrum. With normal lighting, the muscles in the iris are slightly tense all the time. Strip lighting or fluorescent tube lighting is in varying degrees harmful to the eyes. A full-spectrum 'tube' has gone halfway to helping. However, because of the highly responsive vapour, the AC electricity current still leaves us with the unavoidable flicker. Until this is completely corrected, one should not be subjected to this light for any length of time. To correct this, we now have an electronic ballast (*see page 73*).

The Hygeia pure light lamp offers a relaxing illumination while also producing a clear, true light. The actual colour of the light relaxes the eyes while conventional light creates tension.

Those who read, write, sew, embroider or do any colour work in the long winter evenings will soon learn to appreciate this lamp. It is fitted with a dimmer switch that not only allows the light to be gently controlled, but conserves the bulbs and causes no shock to the user.

The Colour Space Illuminator

Do we always need to be in a given illumination which we cannot alter or can we think of another colour to be surrounded by? This question was raised in the early years of our research and through it the colour

Figure 6.6: (From left to right) The colour space Illuminator and the pure light lamp (*see Resources, page 123*).

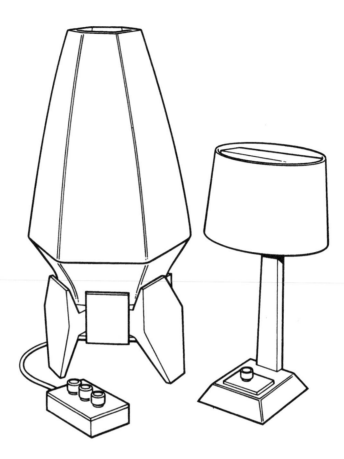

space illuminator was born. This is a lamp with colours that can be changed and mixed according to the wish of the user (*see Figure 6.6*).

The colour space illuminator is not only a beautiful object with infinite colour and brightness changes, but it is also a means by which the owner can benefit in health.

The lamp creates an atmosphere for massage, conversation or listening to music; a happy light as a general background or a soothing one for children who have difficulties sleeping.

Blue is used for calming and lowering blood pressure, the relief of asthma and general relaxation; violet for feeling uplifted; orange when depressed; red for energy and for raising blood pressure.

Green is the only light that is excluded because we feel that it is not a safe colour in the hands of the untrained person.

It is recommended that the actual use of this instrument for therapy is about 3 x 15–20 minutes per week, and that during this time no other activity should be undertaken. One should be either dressed completely in white or undressed.

Practical Exercise: The colour-silk treatment

How about treating yourself to a wonderful experience?

Undress and lie down in a light, warm bedroom with music of your choice playing quietly in the background.

Select one of the colours of the rainbow in the form of a beautiful full-length silk and cover your whole body with it. It is important that you use a pure natural fibre such as cotton, wool or silk. The very best material is silk.

Stay in this position for at least 20 minutes, allowing yourself to listen to the music and to daydream. You might also like to use one of the meditations from Chapter 1. (These are available on tape from Hygeia Studios, *see Resources*).

Transmitting Colour

A fully trained colour practitioner is able to broadcast a treatment to a patient. This has proven to be successful because the spine chart that has been made for a person acts as a communicator of very special energy transmission.

When radio waves were discovered, it became possible to send sound waves over a radius of ever greater distances to any receiver from a transmitter. We now take this fact for granted and use it everywhere in the world; for peaceful, military and medical purposes.

In that band of frequencies, at a higher rate, we break into the colour range of the electromagnetic spectrum. Within it are contained X-rays and, much higher up still, radium waves.

We can transmit colour not only through the TV network but also from a human transmitter to a human receiver. Colour therapy acts in this way. The human instrument learns how to transmit and receive accurate information between the therapist and the patient. Colour is then transmitted by way of light through high-quality filters after a diagnostic spine chart has been made. Through the making of this chart, some colours are transmitted to the patient. Treatment with the patient present and absent work hand in hand.

Some of the conditions that we can treat in the above way are migraine, asthma, stress, AIDS, cancer, inflammatory conditions, autism, mental, emotional and metabolic problems. It must be remembered, however, that colour therapy, like all medical treatment, can only be successful if the patient (a) comes to us in good time and (b) wants to cooperate and is willing to change their general lifestyle. This may include thought (mental activity), feelings (emotions), diet and the physical daily rhythms of the day.

We are all apt to neglect part of ourselves, sometimes for such long periods that disease can enter into our system. If we do not communicate with ourselves, we find that some of our functions go into recession. Many diseases can be caused by interference with human functions. Epilepsy can be caused by strobe lights and autism by a malfunction in the administration of a general anaesthetic. This need not mean that the medical application is wrong, only that the individual person has reacted in a special way according to their own life patterns and no one can be blamed.

We colour therapists claim no cures but are thankful when we find that improvements have occurred through our treatment.

Scanning

Scanning a patient is one of the most powerful types of healing. It was used in ancient temple rituals, but with the advent of the mechanical and machine age much of this knowledge has been lost.

To be able to develop the sensitivity of our own instruments, our bodies, we must be aware that we are composed of the spiritual, the soul and the physical bodies; all of these are incorporated into us as human beings. This acknowledgement is really important as we develop our being more and more and it must be from this viewpoint that one welcomes a patient.

Furthermore, we are also an aura being, an etheric being and a sensual being. The aura field, the most sensitive field, not yet visible to many, carries for us the energies which cause our body to be well or not so well. The etheric body (much smaller than the aura) is close to the physical body of flesh and blood. It carries the response mechanism from our physical body into the life body, which is highly charged spiritually, magnetically and electrically.

Practical Exercise

Another method of working with colour is with stained glass and quartz crystals. Place a stained-glass filter over a small lamp. This needs to be designed so that a good airflow is incorporated into it for cooling. Good-quality stained glass is very expensive and very easily broken by heat.

Place the coloured filter of your choice onto the lamp and then place the quartz crystal on top of the filter. The crystal will now be saturated with your chosen colour.

The crystal needs to remain on the filter for at least 20 minutes. After this interval of time, you can place the solarized crystal on to any part of your body where you feel the colour that you have chosen is needed. This part of your body will gently absorb the crystal-colour energy.

For scanning, the patient is asked to wear natural fibres, such as cotton, silk or wool, and to be dressed in white. If they are not dressed in white then a gown is provided for them.

The therapist scans the patient's energy fields, sensing colour, heat and magnetism. In this way they can usually tell where there are any deficiencies in the organism of the person. The colour healing that follows can be very powerful.

As we grow more and more aware, so we will become conscious of new uses for colour. We must remember that all outer work, both in science and in art, must eventually be brought into the inner mind and become not only a factual memory but also a part of our own being.

In all the efforts you make to maintain your health, you must remember that here, on this planet, we are subject to the five original elements. The first is earth (green), the matter on which we base, and indeed hold together, our liquid state. This state is the second element, water (blue). The third element is our warmth body, which is related to fire (red); the fourth, our gaseous body, which is air (yellow). The given colours for these elements go back to the original teachings of Hippocrates in the fifth century BC. However, according to the work of Rudolph Steiner there is a fifth element that is essential to life and is called ether (violet). It is contained in all the other four (it is the means by which they are alive) and is also an element in its own right. When we work on our health, it is very helpful to see these elements as actual beings as it can help as to visualize the way in which the energy of the elements works. In the next chapter, therefore, we shall examine how to work with these beings, ourselves and the vast cosmic beings known as angels.

Chapter 7

Elements, Humans and Angels

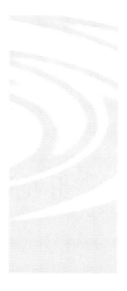

Each soul is potentially divine.
The goal is to manifest this divinity within by
controlling nature, external and internal:
Do this either by work, or worship or psychic
control, or philosophy. By one, or more, or all
of these and be free.
This is the whole of religion, doctrines or dogmas,
or rituals, or books, or temples, or forms, are but
of secondary details

Swami Vivekananda, Raja Yoga

(Advaita Ashrarna S Dehli, Calcutta 14)

magine a figure of eight with the five elements – earth, water, fire, air and ether (*see pages 93–4*) – in the bottom loop and the divine or angelic hierarchies in the top loop. The human race sits where the lines of loops cross and it is our role to unite the two: we were given dominion over the elements so we could be the translators between these two different realms. Somehow, over the course of millennia, we have forgotten how to communicate with them and in so doing have lost touch with ourselves, with the elements and with the realm of the divine. In short, we have disturbed the universal flow of energy.

Although children are born into this world with an innate ability to communicate with this energy, they do not often get confirmation of what they bring with them from the invisible worlds. Sadly, because children are so impressionable, they soon forget this wisdom. This is largely due to education, for in this present age our society is focused on technology and our education reflects this. By and large it is this technological ambition that is turning us into a race that is unable to think holistically; it is blurring our understanding of the vast coherence between all things and that knowledge may eventually slip out of our collective consciousness altogether.

Most of us are unaware that behind the whole of the visible world there are invisible energies allowing the visible world to appear. According to ancient mystics, these cosmic–galactic fields are the source of the spiritual intentions for this planet, including the role we have to play on it. Unfortunately, most of us do not understand these spiritual intentions, or have forgotten them completely, and neglect the part we have to play. In order to heal ourselves and the planet we will have to re-educate ourselves and our children.

The Elements and Kingdoms of Nature

The five elements are earth, water, fire, air and ether, and the three kingdoms of nature are mineral, plant and animal. We can also class these in terms of five elemental worlds – mineral, liquid, warmth, gaseous, kingdom of minerals – and four kingdoms of nature – plants, animals, humans, etheric energy. Each of these has an associated colour.

ELEMENTS

Mineral world	Earth	Green
Liquid world	Water	Blue
Warmth world	Fire	Red
Gaseous world	Air	Yellow
Kingdom of minerals	Crystals	White/magenta (delta rhythms)

KINGDOMS OF NATURE

Plants	Plant	Gold (zeta rhythms)
Animals	Animal	Indigo (alpha rhythms)
Humans	Human	Multicolour (beta rhythms)
Etheric energy	Ether	Violet

When we are very excited, our brains pulse at around 34 pulses per second. This is called beta plus. When we are relaxed this decreases to around 21 times per second, known as beta. These typical pulse levels are not normally experienced as colour, although in actual fact they are multicoloured.

The different kingdoms of nature all pulse at different rates and if we can control our brain pulse speed we can reach higher states of communication with them. Meditation is an ideal way to do this. If we can slow our brain pulses to 13 per second, called alpha, our minds will become peaceful and we will experience the calmness that the colour blue offers. This is the level of animal pulses and you will find that animals will immediately trust and cooperate with you if your mind is in this state. Zeta is the state of plants and they pulse only eight times per second. You should take care entering this state without an experienced instructor. In a zeta state you experience the colour gold and people become almost transparent. If you can train your mind to enter zeta before harvesting or cutting plants, the plant will remain calm and not withdraw its energies from the leaves or fruit. Delta pulses about five times per second and you should not attempt to enter this state without an experienced teacher or very careful instructions, otherwise you may panic. While you can reach this state in a deep sleep, in a super-aware state it can paralyse you. In this state you experience a brilliant white with a hint of magenta. This is the realm of the mineral kingdom.

Drugs

Some hallucinogenic drugs can slow brain pulses to zeta (drugs that slow the brain below seven pulses per second are lethal), but they interfere with the communication between the ego, astral, etheric and physical bodies. They are also addictive and render people incapable of being the master of their own minds. Meditation is a much safer, more efficient way to slow down the brain pulses as it teaches you to free the mind in a self aware and responsible way (*see page 98 for instructions on how to meditate*).

Elemental Beings

It will also help us communicate with the elements if we accept that they are not just matter. Just as we live in our bodies, so, too, beings live in the energies of earth, water, fire and air and make these elements alive. Normally we cannot see these creatures, but when we are ready, at the moment of asking if they really exist, they will reveal themselves, little by little. Although their energy is always the same, their appearance cannot be described as such – everybody sees them slightly differently. In days gone by wise men and women could see these beings locked in the molecules of the elements. They are as powerful as the very mighty angels and eternal masters in the invisible spiritual worlds, with whom we are more familiar. The names of these beings are inherited from the ancient texts of the Greeks.

The element of earth, the whole of the mineral world, is subdivided into crystals, metals and sedimentary rock, and the beings locked within are known as Gnomes. Gnomes give the minerals solidity.

93

Great areas of our planet are covered in water, be it in the form of springs, lakes, rivers or oceans. The beings residing inside water are called Undines. Salamanders are the beings that are responsible for the warmth world – the glow that is inside the mountains and apparent in the heat of fire and light. And within the molecules of air, the breath of life and all gaseous energy, are beings called the Sylphs.

The fifth element, ether – also known as the kingdom of etheric energy – penetrates the other four elements, giving them life. It is the force within all things, responsible for the growth of crystals, plants, animals and humans. It is the realm of the masters and its associated colour is violet. Ether is a great healer and behind it stand invisible cosmic rays. The beings inside this element have many names, none of which adequately conveys their power and energy and puts limits on their potential. It is therefore appropriate that, ultimately, they have no one set name.

The elemental beings in ether are waiting for us to choose the right way to see the other elements beyond their clinical and material components, and find freedom from division. They are waiting for us to find unity in duality, for neither men nor women could exist alone. We need to communicate again with the beings in these five elements in order to heal ourselves and the planet. Only then can the universal energy flow freely through the figure of eight.

In an age where scientific proof is everything, it is often difficult for us to conceive of these beings. Yet there is so much in the world that remains unexplained, particularly in the physics of the very small.

If we can, at this point, call these unexplained riddles the elemental beings, the invisible forces within minerals, water, fire and air, we may be led into areas where new answers can be found.

Certainly colour leads us into a part of such explanations. Concentration, too, leads by the same principle of polarity (duality) into relaxation, time off, not thinking, not being filled with a content; just as we need sleep after waking. A short period of concentration during research (being awake), followed by a period of absolute relaxation, forgetting instead of remembering, is a principle of Rudolf Steiner's teaching. Make your mind free of thoughts, concepts and ideas; listen, otherwise you will not hear; look, otherwise you will not see. We need to apply this idea of opposites to every moment in our daily work. Let the fear to forget dissolve into the trust to remember. When you relax, ask the angels and the elemental beings to give you the information which you require now.

To receive such messages, you have to let go, relax and meditate. Relax and then receive healing. Relax and then be aware.

The Elemental Energy Patterns

In all the endless patterns of this planet and in the souls and hearts of people, we will never find two identical beings or events. However, there is an underlying principle which can be considered a kind of blueprint: a form encloses an area and into this come forces which want to enter and forces which want to go out. Here we have the duality of life: breathing in, breathing out; sleeping and waking; activity and passivity; gravity and levity; colour and complementary colour.

A very fast 'aura'-like energy is around all the living kingdoms, whether these are small or large or the whole. This energy can be perceived by those who can 'see' the energy fields, the aura.

All the elements – earth, water, fire and air – and also the mineral plant, animal and human kingdoms have a kind of 'breathing' pattern. The denser the substance, the faster the inflow energy becomes. Plants have a great amount of inflow but some outflow when measured against the mineral world. When ultimately a person arrives at the stage where they can 'breathe' rhythmically in and out, then there arises the state of consciousness that creates awareness. The more a manifested energy can breathe out, the more the consciousness can develop. The principle is that by way of the outflow an energy field is expanded and a counterflow is the inevitable result. This

Figure 7.1: The mineral element. The mineral world has a very fast inflow energy, marked by the arrows pointing inwards, and almost no outflow energy; that is the reason why most people call it dead. However, nothing is dead on this planet.

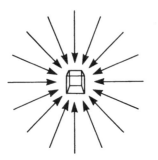

may become unbearable to those who cannot manage to handle the information received in this way and many end up in mental hospitals where drugs and ECT are then used to control their input. Most, indeed, are then 'vegetables'. (*See also* José Silva, *Mind Control*.)

The Element of Earth

The very, very small creatures which we can behold in the mineral world are the Gnomes. These are concealed in the molecule of each cell. The atom's existence is due to the neutron and proton circling around in space and creating the energy that we call 'atom'. This again demonstrates the same principle. Call the proton orange and the neutron blue and you will be able to experience this in colour.

The Element of Water

Undines live in every single moisture particle. There are millions, like the Gnomes, in an invisible space. Where is the limit on either side? Out there in space or in here in the minute particle?

The Element of Fire

The warmth of the fire element also causes light, but that light and warmth have perhaps lost the quality of love. This element now burns too hot and is often impure. It dazzles and hurts our eyes. The Salamander beings are tiny flecks of fire which are there to cleanse and illuminate. Because of the lack of human communica-tion, they have grown estranged and in their isolation cry out, often in anger, saying, 'Hey, you, I am also here, take notice of me.' Like neglected and ignored children, they often play naughty tricks until someone notices them. Although, if they are kindly, lovingly approached they will, little by little, aid the human race again and shine brightly. They will no longer burn but create warmth so that pure life can again evolve.

Figure 7.2: The water element. The water element still has a very fast inflow of energy but does give out some of this energy, especially the very fine etheric energy; the arrows indicate its energy exchange.

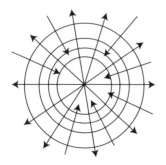

Figure 7.3: The fire element. Fire energy is a very special element. It is said that Prometheus stole it from the Gods on Olympus and gave it to man against the wishes of the gods.

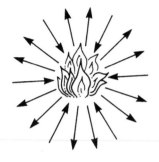

The Element of Air

With the element of air, the very breath of life, the duality of inhaling and exhaling was known to be the dance of the Sylphs.

The human race has grossly misused this element by way of pollution, filling up the space of life where the ether could live, the prana, the energy of spiritual angelic beings. Because of toxic gases, less and less constructive communication is being transmitted and the Sylphs, like all other elemental beings, are rebelling. They even withdraw and hide away. Human thanks must be given for their service and human protection and blessing must return. We have to pour in love again, to give it freely because we wish to do so. Then communication will again be possible. Human souls who offer this new recognition to this element will return to health. Likewise, in places where a lack of air may prove fatal, call upon the Sylphs with thanks, blessing and love, and help will be given to restore life because we have reunited ourselves with these creatures.

We should also link all of the elementals back to the angelic world and the great spiritual beings such as the Buddha, the Christ, Jehovah and Allah. This will enable them to speak to each other again. Man will then have learnt the languages of both these great kingdoms and can take up his predestined place as the selfless and

Figure 7.4: The air element. The element of air, the breath of life, has indeed its own breath. it breathes in to the time of two and out to the time of three. It is filled with etheric energy, which is also known as prana.

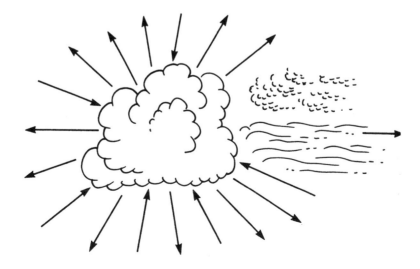

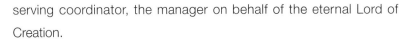

serving coordinator, the manager on behalf of the eternal Lord of Creation.

Communication Meditations

The following six meditations are to help you tap in to each of the five elements: earth, water, fire, air and ether. The sixth meditation, the Exchange Breathing, will help you to connect to all five elements at once and stabilize your energy field. I always find that this is my students' favourite meditation as it leaves them with a great sense of calm, well-being and balance. These are all perfectly safe meditations so you can do them alone even if you are new to meditation.

Do not try to memorize the text for each meditation. Read it through slowly and let the words inspire you to create your own dialogue. Don't try to remember every word as you will stop mid-meditation and freeze your thoughts if you forget a word and this can be very disorientating. If you prefer, you can ask a friend, a loved one or spiritual guide to read out the text and lead you through the meditation; alternatively, you could read it out loud into a tape recorder and play it back. The most important thing is to relax into the meditation, to visualize the colours and to try and dissolve yourself into the relevant element.

Preparation

Clean and declutter the room in which you intend to meditate to dispel any stagnant energy. Switch on the answerphone and ensure you will not be disturbed for at least an hour. Keep a blanket nearby in case you get cold.

When you are ready, light a candle or burn a few drops of your favourite essential oil. When you light the candle you can hold it upright and send out a thought for a loved one, person in need or a specific purpose. Sit cross-legged on the floor or on a stool. If possible, keep your back upright throughout the meditation to help create a link between the universe and the centre of the Earth.

If you are on your own you may want to call upon the angels, God, Buddha or spirit of the Earth to guide and protect you, depending on your personal beliefs. Alternatively, adapt the protection meditation below, substituting 'God' for a spiritual guide you can relate to, be it Allah, Buddha, Christ, Gaia, Ganesh or Jehovah. It is known as the St Patrick's Breastplate and dates from AD 435. Say it slowly, pausing for about five seconds between each line.

God is behind me,
God is below me,
God is at my left side,
God is at my right side,
God is before me,
God is above me,
God is within me.
God is in the darkness of my thinking,
God is in the light of my thinking,
God is in the colours of my aura,
God is in the sounds of my speaking,
God is in the form of my body,
God is the overlord of all creation.

If you have asked someone to be your guide through the meditation, you may want them to begin with a dedication of their intent to help you. They can say a few words spontaneously or they may wish to read a poem, prayer or passage from a spiritual text. I find this dedication always works well.

MY DEDICATION

Gracious Divine Beings, in all my communications with my fellow humans I transmit your healing powers. My intentions are to be the Channel of love, purity and beauty. Grant today that I am in the right place, at the right time for the right action. I wish to be your helper in healing. I ask to be restored at the end of the day with your etheric life force.

Amen

Ideally, your guide should be an experienced master or the tutor in charge. This is because the person must have enough conscious-ness to be aware what stage anyone under their guidance has reached, otherwise the meditator's mind can go out of control and mental illness may ensue. However, if an experienced guide is not available, a loved one whose intentions are pure will normally guide you just as safely through the meditations.

When you have completed the meditation, it is important to declare it is over. This could be through saying something as simple as, 'This is from my heart', or 'Amen' or 'So be it'. Choose the words that you feel comfortable with. If you are with a guide, they can bring you back to the here and now with another simple meditation (*see page 114*).

The Earth (Mineral) Kingdom

Relax and let go of all your daily concerns. Let the instrument, your body, go into calmness, peace and absolute harmony. With each exhalation, make sure that you are letting go of all tension.

Let the bright multicolours in your busy mind disappear. Now wait for a deep blue to appear before your inner eye. Relax even more, allowing the golden light to dissolve all the petty pictures which you are still trying to hold before your mind. Think of a white, beautifully illuminated energy with a very fine, almost invisible magenta colour toned into a pure resurrected red. Red, the colour of the Father energy. The centre, the awareness, now turning into the energy of the son and daughter, the energy of love, a rose quartz colour.

Be thankful for this moment. Bless this time and love the communication that you are about to receive. Be open in safety. Your guide is aware that you are being protected.

You stand on the earth, a firm rock upon which we can depend for safety. We cannot be inside this rock as it is too dense, solid and hard. Yet, with our mind, we can slip into this dense, very compact space.

This is from my heart.

The Water Kingdom

Relax and let go of all your daily concerns. Let the instrument, your body, go into calmness, peace and absolute harmony. With each exhalation, make sure that you are letting go of all tension.

Let the bright multicolours in your busy mind disappear. Now wait for a deep blue to appear before your inner eye. Relax even more, allowing the golden light to dissolve all the petty pictures which you are still trying to hold before your mind. Think of a white, beautifully illuminated energy with a very fine, almost invisible magenta colour toned into a pure resurrected red. Red, the colour of the Father energy. The centre, the awareness, now turning into the energy of the son and daughter, the energy of love, a rose quartz colour.

Be thankful for this moment. Bless this time and love the communication that you are about to receive. Be open in safety. Your guide is aware that you are being protected.

Water. The water of life. The chalice filled from the fountain where water is carrying the life, the reflected light and the caressing love.

Water is the home of the Undines. These water elementals are the carriers of etheric living energy which once came down from the great cosmic ether and anchored itself in water, to heal, to cleanse, to refresh body, soul and spirit.

The Undine kingdom is present in the energies in the warm state when fire (Salamanders) play with the Undines and create in their play a warm, life-enhancing moisture that we can breathe in, healing our bodies with an enhanced breath of life. See this chalice lifted up to your lips. Take into your senses its scent, its fragrance. The two energies of water Undines and fire Salamanders create the third energy of living fragrance. As they dance, they create new forms and the new forms give new life. See on the floor where they have been, the traces left. These are like seeds lying in the fertile earth. The Gnomes are taking care of them. We stand high up and look down on to this wonderful dance floor. As we look, we can see that the seeds all sprout and, behold, what wonderful patterns are now visible.

In a creative way we wonder. As we wonder, we are already creating new ideas on how to follow the dance, to learn the new dance. We now thank the Undines for their inspiration. Out of the silence we hear a sound, a singing. The music of the Undines mingles with the music of the angels, the music of the spheres. The singing changes into harmonies not hitherto heard by us. This is a direct result of our humble effort to communicate as best we know how.

We are learning, we are beginning to interpret our own, however incomplete, speech with both the elementals and the angels.

We are now using the circle of light and the cross of light in the circle of light as a golden key to close the centres of higher perception securely: the crown, the brow, the throat, the heart, the solar plexus, the sacral and the base energy centre (*see page 114*).

Remember where you started the meditation, the room, the house, and when you are ready you may slowly open your eyes and be fully returned.

This is from my heart.

The Fire Kingdom

Relax and let go of all your daily concerns. Let the instrument, your body, go into calmness, peace and absolute harmony. With each exhalation, make sure that you are letting go of all tension.

Let the bright multicolours in your busy mind disappear. Now wait for a deep blue to appear before your inner eye. Relax even more, allowing the golden light to dissolve all the petty pictures which you are still trying to hold before your mind. Think of a white, beautifully illuminated energy with a very fine, almost invisible magenta colour toned into a pure resurrected red. Red, the colour of the Father energy. The centre, the awareness, now turning into the energy of the son and daughter, the energy of love, a rose quartz colour.

Be thankful for this moment. Bless this time and love the communication that you are about to receive. Be open in safety. Your guide is aware that you are being protected.

Try and see a cube, a space which is like a tiny room with four walls, a floor and a ceiling all of the same size. Look inside, imagining it to be on the palm of your hand. You see thousands of even smaller cubes inside this tiny room. In each there are uncountable little Gnomes, all busy creating and maintaining this mineral substance.

Now it has become alive in your mind's eye. It is no longer just matter, it is living matter which is at all times ready to serve you. It will serve you even more if you think how it needs your thanks for being, just being. It can change when you bless it and love it. The Gnomes will then be at your command and prevent any mishaps. You can tell them to make this matter strong, to hold it together in the way that you wish it to be, so that it can serve you. Now you have to be aware of the reason for this. Why do you need this matter which has been built to serve you? Are you using it for the service of others or is it being used for your own selfish gain? Examine your motives. You can only truly be thankful for this matter, shaped for your use, if it is used in a way that can help those who are as yet not as awake as you are.

To be awake means to know and to employ the knowledge in such a way that it serves those whom you meet.

Now you can bless it and the Gnomes can become aware of your gift. To them this blessing is similar to your daily bread. Then send to them love, because you know that in the end this is the most precious gift that you can offer.

In the peace and stillness you can now communicate. Be silent for a while. Listen, let go of any thoughts, just listen, listen with your other, inner ears. At present we have lost this capacity and it will take some time before we again reach this level of hearing. Try to listen, really listen. When we learn a new language, it takes some time to really know it. We first have to learn, to understand the actual speaking. This is always very difficult. Have patience.

Now turn your inner gaze to the vast spaces outside of the tiny room which you hold in your hand. Think how you could tell the angels what you have experienced. Again, to begin with, you cannot form any words as these are of the earth. Just look, and you will begin to see with your inner eyes. Allow all the conventional pictures of angels to go away, to dissolve into a vast open room, a hall where the walls, ceiling and floor are too far away to see. A very small part of the great angelic being is there. The whole of this inconceivable great being we cannot as yet comprehend. A great sound of deepest singing, ringing, fills the hall. There is no time or space. You are alone, but not lonely. No one else is here, but all are here. There is a fulfilled energy and we can only add wonder, awe and reverence. Can we take the thanks, the blessings and the love that we communicated to the Gnomes and lay them down in this enormous place? Yes, we can.

The singing changes into harmonies not hitherto heard by us. This is a direct result of our humble effort to communicate as best we know how. (*See The Book of Sound Therapy* by Olivia Dewhurst-Maddock.)

We are learning, we are beginning to interpret our own, however incomplete, speech with both the elementals and the angels.

We are now using the circle of light and the cross of light in the circle of light as a golden key to close the centres of higher perception securely: the crown, the brow, the throat, the heart, the solar plexus, the sacral and the base energy centre (*see page 114*).

Remember where you started the meditation, the room, the house, and when you are ready, you may open your eyes and be fully returned.

This is from my heart.

The Air Kingdom

Relax and let go of all your daily concerns. Let the instrument, your body, go into calmness, peace and absolute harmony. With each exhalation make sure that you are letting go of all tension.

Let the bright multicolours in your busy mind disappear. Now wait for a deep blue to appear before your inner eye. Relax even more, allowing the golden light to dissolve all the petty pictures which you are still trying to hold before your mind. Think of a white, beautifully illuminated energy with a fine, almost invisible magenta colour toned into a pure resurrected red. Red, the colour of the Father energy. The centre, the awareness, now turning into the energy of the son and daughter, the energy of love, a rose quartz colour.

Be thankful for this moment. Bless this time and love the communication that you are about to receive. Be open in safety. Your guide is aware that you are being protected.

A beautiful garden lies before you and you enter this garden by walking across the meadow. Countless flowers are close to your feet. Shrubs and trees are on either side of you. Stand still, wait and look more closely and absorb what is surrounding you. As you stand there, it is important that you feel no wish to hurry. You sit down on the soft grass. Peace and relaxation overcome you and a beautiful blue light dawns inside your third eye. This light spreads all over you, enabling you to relax completely into the environment. The blue slowly changes into a calm gold light. It makes the space that you are in appear larger. A very gentle breeze moves your hair, caresses your skin and you become aware that your breath is very slow and very deep. What is this air that you are using in order to live? If it keeps you alive, it in itself must be alive. You ask, 'What are you, air?'

Out of this stillness comes a whisper: 'I was part of God. I am all around you. As you need me, so I need you. We are intertwined. You are able to change me because I can only partly help you. The other part of me that you cannot use is the part used by the trees, shrubs and flowers. You can help to reunite me with the wholeness which I once was.

'What is it that I can do for you? Have you got a name?'

'Yes, I do have a name, but firstly, I am not able to be a single being. I am actually we, so you talk to all of us.'

'Please tell me then what you call yourselves, all of you.

'We are known as the Sylphs, the elemental spirits of the air.'

'How can I be of help to you?'

'Take us back to the great energy of God and the angels. You can talk to the angels but we can no longer do this. You humans have come between us and the original wholeness of us. Talk to the angels and tell them about our state now.'

'How have you changed? Why are you saying this about your state now?'

'You took the first step to freedom, to become separate from God when you took the fruit from the Tree of Knowledge. You now know the secrets of God, but you have forgotten the life, the Tree of Life. The breath of air is no longer the same since you used your knowledge. The air that we are now is heavy with wrongly used knowledge. You cannot change this back to the living state unless you change a part of yourselves. You humans have forgotten in all your great knowledge that gratitude, blessing and love are all part of the purity of life. The living breath of air needs to be regained. When you come to us with the three great gifts of love, thanks and blessing, we will help you to achieve this task.

'Tell the trees and the plants that you will give to them the part of the air, the part of us, that you are unable to use. If you become a mediator between us and the angels, you will be a creator of a new air, a new breath of life. This new air and breath of life will start a new cycle because you have changed us. Unless you help us, all the air must die, also us and you. Must we all die? No. If you can follow the path of love, blessing and gratitude, we will all have created a new and very beautiful breath of love, much more alive than it was at the beginning.'

'Can I see you Sylphs?'

'Yes, you can if you can deeply relax. Relax, and now, what can you see?'

'Is what I see correct? Are you completely invisible, transparent beings? Are there uncountable numbers of you in the tiniest space?'

'So you can see us?'

'Yes, I think I can.'

'Yes, you have now seen us. We dance around and within you. We also dance around and within all plants. But, it is only you that can make the new air. Only you who can redeem us out of the present state where we are captive in this heavy air. Change yourself and you will change the universe for all eternity to come.'

We must have sat here for a long time talking to the Sylphs. We now need to go about our daily work knowing that we will work each day with the changes which we have to make. We will thank, we will bless, we will love the Sylphs and we will also talk to the angels about them.

Now you have found the little garden where you can communicate with the Sylphs and the angels. You are now taking up your task and you go into the world of substance where you count, weigh and measure, but now you add the new ingredients of thanks, blessing and love.

The singing changes into harmonies not hitherto heard by us. This is a direct result of our humble effort to communicate as best we know how.

We are learning, we are beginning to interpret our own, however incomplete, speech with both the elementals and the angels.

We are now using the circle of light and the cross of light in the circle of light as a golden key to close the centres of higher perception securely: the crown, the brow, the throat, the heart, the solar plexus, the sacral and the base energy centre (*see page 114*).

Remember where you started the meditation, the room, the house and when you are ready you may slowly open your eyes and be fully returned.

This is from my heart.

The Etheric Energy of Life

Relax and let go of all your daily concerns. Let the instrument, your body, go into calmness, peace and absolute harmony. With each exhalation, make sure that you are letting go of all tension.

Let the bright multicolours in your busy mind disappear. Now wait for a deep blue to appear before your inner eye. Relax even more, allowing the golden light to dissolve all the petty pictures which you are still trying to hold before your mind. Think of a white, beautifully illuminated energy with a very ftne, almost invisible magenta colour toned into a pure resurrected red. Red, the colour of the Father energy. The centre, the awareness, now turning into the energy of the son and daughter, the energy of love, a rose quartz colour.

Be thankful for this moment. Bless this time and love the communication that you are about to receive. Be open in safety. Your guide is aware that you are being protected.

We are going into the night, out into the vast space which is without borders, but we are very safe. There are beautiful 'wings' of protection around us.

The darkness is not really dark but it has the colour of a deep indigo-violet; it is warm, it is full of beauty. Sparkling around us are gold stars which make such wonderful patterns that we cannot yet find any repeats or pictures that we recognize.

We become aware of a presence of energy that seems to have the form of very fine and noble features. Through this wonderful deep colour of the indigo-violet shines an image created out of light. Not a strong light, not a blinding light, but a gentle and yet very clear light that makes out the features of a most elevated being. We recognize in it the perfect image of a spiritual being who is eternally young and yet beautifully mature. We are drawn to it to be united with it. We sense that it is part of us and yet a being of energy that is far more alive than we are. Part of this life we recognize within us and it is like a mirror that reflects the perfect life force without.

It is as if we are now seeing an unending ocean of life force which breathes, like waves, in and out with a rhythm of eternity. The gold, the light, the deep indigo-violet are reflected in it and have an eternal everlasting beauty. As we now look down at our own feet, standing very close to this ocean, we can see our own image and we can see that we seem to bear a very close likeness to this great being; as if we were just one cell of it. We are asked to accept a part of this eternal energy so that we can become a part of this great wholeness. We seem to drink, as though it were out of a chalice, the energy that is now all around us. As we accept this wonderfully refreshing, renewing, reviving, rejuvenating drink, we begin to see ourselves as part of this life force that is eternal.

We look up and see once more the immensely wonderful image, and hands which seem to offer it to us, which stretch out towards us. In gratitude we accept this gift. We hear the words, 'Take this, close it into your heart and guard it so that life never ebbs for you. Accept, transform and release so that you are a pure channel of communication between the angels and the elemental beings. You can become an eternally well, flowing being like we are.'

Now we are returning to the place where we started, the room or space where we started our meditation.

We are now using the circle of light and the cross of light in the circle of light as a golden key to close the centres of higher perception securely: the crown, the brow, the throat, the heart, the solar plexus, the sacral and the base energy centre.

This is from my heart.

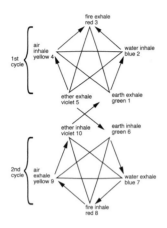

Figure 7.5: Exchange breathing.

Exchange Breathing

This is a special meditation for people who have difficulty stabilizing their lives. You will also find it helpful if you have problems sleeping. It will reconnect you to the five elements. It is a ten-part visualization that takes you through two cycles of five (*see Figure 7.5*). Each cycle works through the five elements and you either breathe in their purifying energies to cleanse your body and mind or breathe out into them to release your own negative energies. Each element has an associated colour and it is important to imagine breathing out or into the appropriate colour. As with the other meditations, don't try to memorize this one word for word if you are doing it on your own; instead, absorb the essence of the meditation and improvise.

Part 1: Earth Exhale

COLOUR: GREEN

On a warm summer afternoon we are lying on a rock, covered with moss, warmed by the sun. The Gnomes know that we are there and start talking to us. 'Breathe out all your tensions and toxins and waste cells into the rock. We will turn them into useful energy; they are our raw material. Breathe out into the earth.'

Do this slowly three times and with gratitude.

Now there are spaces within our body and we tell the angels, the Seraphim, what the Gnomes have told us. A flood of peace and relaxation comes over us. We feel that we are out of time and space; minutes become hours and hours become minutes. We thank the angels and the Gnomes and take seven normal breaths to end this first part of the meditation.

Part 2: Water Inhale

COLOUR: BLUE

We are walking into a beautiful green valley. It is morning. At the end of the valley there are rocks, over which a waterfall is tumbling. The Undines invite us to go and stand under this fresh, clear mountain water and breathe in three times. Do this three times and feel how your body is refreshed and purified. Say 'thank you' to the Undines.

Angels can now penetrate this fine new water element. We have reconnected elementals and angels and we thank both of them and take seven normal breaths to end this second part of the meditation.

Part 3: Fire Exhale

COLOUR: RED

We are now walking into a grotto and there is burning flame of fire. The elementals of fire, the Salamanders, are saying: 'This, our fire, is the fire that cleanses you of all negative thoughts, fears and doubts. Breathe out into these flames three times and allow yourself to listen to your heart. Let your mind be purified and let us burn away all your petty annoyances.'

Breathe out three times into the flames as instructed.

We promise the Salamanders we will take their advice to the angels, who are now here as angels of light. We thank both elementals and angels and take seven normal breaths to end this third part of the meditation.

Part 4: Air Inhale

COLOUR: YELLOW

We are in a garden on a sunny, summer morning and see the beautiful green leaves. 'Breathe in what we breathe out,' we hear the Sylphs saying to us.

We breathe in and out and the Sylphs are so happy to receive our exhalation.

'We use your exhaled breath to give to the plants as important raw material,' they say.

Breathe in three times and say 'thank you'.

Once we have done this, we feel that we have made new space inside our lungs and have breathed in much more than just air. We thank the Sylphs and the hierarchy of angels and as before take seven breaths to end this fourth part of the meditation.

Part 5: Ether Exhale

COLOUR: VIOLET

The realm that we now enter is new to us. We have not much knowledge of it. It is a deep violet-magenta colour that we have always called black, but it is not black. In this etheric realm are all the forces which renew our own life force. Here are the beings we call God, angels and the very highly accomplished masters who have successfully learned all the bitter lessons which the contracted energies of matter have taught us. These angels tell us to breathe out into this divine space so that we are refreshed and our etheric energy is renewed.

Breathe out three times and trust that all will be well when we have been allowed to sleep well.

Then we say three 'thank you's and take seven quiet breaths before we travel further.

Part 6: Earth Inhale

COLOUR: GREEN

We come down into a cave which is covered with crystals. The Gnomes greet us and say, 'Breathe in as many of our crystals as you need to be strong and well. Yes, breathe in three earth times. This beautiful clear earth has an inner light; the angelic forces have cleared it of all obscure matter. Take three breaths and see your cells shining with transparent light.'

Say, 'Thank you Gnomes and angels,' and go on your way.

Part 7: Water Exhale

COLOUR: BLUE

There is a beautiful river before us and the Undines greet us, 'Step in and lie down in our flowing water. Breathe out all your unwanted fluid and let us work with it for your betterment.'

Breathe out three times.

We are now met by the angels of all the waters. We thank the Undines and the angels three times and step out of the river onto the other side.

Part 8: Fire Inhale

COLOUR: RED

At this point in our journey, we come back to our grotto. The Salamanders have lit one very beautiful flame for us and say, 'Come in and be part of this flame of consciousness and warmth of heart. Breathe in as much of our light and warmth as you wish. Take three breaths of our gift to you!'

We breathe in three times and become warm and full of light and before us stand the angels of light. We thank the Salamanders and angels three times, take seven normal breaths and move on.

Part 9: Air Exhale

COLOUR: YELLOW

In the garden the trees and shrubs stand in the dusk of a peaceful evening. The Sylphs say to us, 'Breathe out into the evening air all your stress and tension.'

Breathe out into the leaves and say 'thank you' three times.

Now, as before, we become aware of the angels of the air and let them know what the Sylphs have told us. Again, we say 'thank you' three times then we take seven breaths in silence before going on to complete the journey.

Part 10: Ether Inhale

COLOUR: VIOLET

Finally, we are asked to step into the deep violet–magenta universe and the highest beings invite us to breathe in our renewed aura and etheric body. 'Breathe in three times,' these highly evolved beings instruct, 'and be aware of our presence according to your will and freely chosen path.'

Thank you, thank you, thank you.

This is from my heart.

Grounding Meditation

In this meditation and the following ones the student in meditation training will be shown graphically the circle of light and the cross of light in the circle of light.

1 The circle is the symbol of surrounding in a protective way; in this case the circle is the colour of gold.
2 The cross is the reminder of being conscious and is almost white with some rose quartz colour in it.
3 The complete symbol is then visualized over each chakra as the meditation closes.

This is vital to bring the student back into the here-and-now world after meditation.

Light and warmth are around us. The inner light and the inner warmth. When we need the help of the Salamanders they can turn cold into warmth and can turn darkness into light.

We are inside a cave; there is at present no light and it is very cold. Relax, let go of any tension. Trust that you are protected and that no harm will come to you.

A tiny spark of light in the distance begins to flicker. It is coming nearer and starts to be a stable, fine light. It now comes closer to us, and little by little, very peacefully burns brighter. The Salamander beings are basically very shy and like to make sure that they are welcome. They respond to love from the hearts of human beings and this protects them. They are also shy towards the elemental beings of water, the Undines, and also shy away from the Sylphs, the elementals of the air. If both of these elementals are very gentle towards the Salamanders, however, they can play together and create surprising effects.

Now the Salamander beings are before you in uncountable numbers. They spread a beautiful light all over the cave. With this light also comes a gentle warmth. Now the cave is a most wonderful place. It is like a hall in a very special palace. Everything shines in a golden colour. The gold of wisdom. Because we have offered love, the response is all around us. We seem to be in the centre of a universal heart that reflects the love we offered and has created this most precious palace for us. All is built out of warmth and light, gentle light, loving warmth.

We say 'thank you' for this beautiful experience, we bless the moment of our vision and we leave forever our love for the Salamanders.

The singing changes into harmonies not hitherto heard by us. This is a direct result of our humble effort to communicate as best we know how.

We are learning, we are beginning to interpret our own, however incomplete, speech with both the elementals and the angels.

We are now using the circle of light and the cross of light in the circle of light as a golden key to close the centres of higher perception securely: the crown, the brow, the throat, the heart, the solar plexus, the sacral and the base energy centre.

Remember where you started the meditation, the room, the house and when you are ready, you may slowly open your eyes and be fully returned.

This is from my heart.

Conclusion

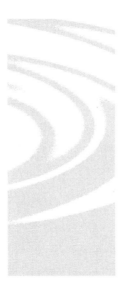

We have examined colour from many points of view: the scientific, which measures, weighs and counts; the spiritual, which can only be appreciated through the human heart; and that of the heart, which knows the truth without needing any scientific proof. You and I have experienced colour and all its energies, both through outward phenomena and through the inner power of visualization.

Life is eternal though it may appear in stages. Life was, is and will be immeasurable forever; that's why it is alive. The art is to translate the information we receive into the words of language or the beauty of art. Perfect art can be like poetry which does not allow only logic to rule; when words are united with other words, they can suddenly change their meaning:

Cuthman: *This is the morning to take the air, flute-clear*
And, like a lutanist, with a hand of wind
Playing the responsive hills, till a long vibration
Spills across the fields, and the chancelled larches
Sing like Lenten choirboys, a green treble;
Playing at last the skylark into rising,

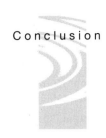

Conclusion

The wintered cuckoo to a bashful stutter.
It is the first day of the year that I've king'd
Myself on the rock, sat myself in the wind:
It was laying my face on gold.

Christopher Fry, *The Boy with a Cart*

Could you also try this using unusual colours and see what they say to each other?

In the chapters of this book I have tried to convey ideas, reality, art, psychic experiences and visualizations which appeal to both the brain and the heart of man.

You may have found some of the ideas difficult. You must, however, allow logic, reason and material reality to mix or communicate with feeling, sensitivity and love. When you do this you will never stop growing.

At first, everything may seem to be overwhelming and so complex that you cannot see the wood for the trees. But then you realize that you are in the wood and that each tree has an individual self to add to the wood. Then you can relax and accept the complexity. In fact it all becomes far simpler and you see that love embraces all and logic divides all. Both need each other to find a way, a way we all tread, thinking we are all alone. Then one day we suddenly arrive in a clearing and find all the others who also thought that they were lost, alone and full of fear and we suddenly recognize each other.

So it is that all the colours make up the rainbow; each colour is individual but also a part of the rainbow.

Finally, each colour is a family of beings within which each individual has the particular hue necessary to make the colour real. Colour is a living medium so sensitive that it is actually affected by the slightest alteration in light. Is it not strange that colour has had to go so long unrecognized as a reality among all the vibrations which are used in science? Its beauty has, perhaps, blinded many, because it is the medium that makes this world such a garden. Yet this beautiful colourful garden is vital to our healing.

119

Fortunately, the true meaning and importance of colour are gradually being recognized. It is as if it is about to be 'crowned' as the supreme being through which life, beauty, energy and harmony are projected to mankind. Perhaps this is the step we finally have to take, now that so much has not really worked. When we finally realize that colour entirely needs to be used in the world of healing, it will become the means by which we can absorb the vibrations that will gently carry life and health back into the discordant structures of modern lifestyles, where so little is beautiful and everything must be practical and useful. Colour combined with other harmonies, such as music and beautiful forms, will bring together the complete spectrum.

Glossary

Aniline
: A chemical dye, very poisonous.

Asthma
: A condition connected to breathing difficulties. Can occur as a result of shock, either mental, emotional or physical.

Autism
: A mental condition that can cause schizophrenia.

Ayurveda
: The original Indian medical practice using colour and gemstones.

Babbitt, Edwin, D.
: (1828–1905). Studied in depth the electromagnetic spectrum and its use in healing, and linked light and colour to universal energies and the divinity of man. *See* Bibliography.

Beesley, Ronald
: (1905–1979). A colour healer with the gift of clairvoyance. *See* Bibliography.

Besant, Annie
: (1847–1933). Member of the Theosophical Society. Studied the Tibetan sacred wisdom and order of the human being.

Byzantine
: A culture that was very prominent from the time of Pythagoras right into the fifth century AD. Arising in the city of Constantinople, its influence stretched into the north Italian cities of Ravenna and Venice, which is shown by the beautiful colours used in their mosaic art. It always had strong connections with Greece.

Camphill Schools
: Educational establishments for the care of mentally handicapped children and adults.

Chagall, Marc	(1887–1985). Born in Russia and studied in Paris. Artist and designer of church windows, for example the Stephans Kirche in Mainz, Germany, his last major work.
Chakra	A Sanskrit word meaning 'wheel'. The chakras are thought to have a connection with endocrine glands in the human body.
Claustrophobia	A condition, mainly mental, of being unable to endure small spaces or being in a crowd. Agoraphobia, the complementary problem, involves being unable to endure too much space without the security of an enclosed room.
Dinshah, P. Ghadiali	(1873–1966). Came from Malaga, New Jersey, USA, and held many honorary degrees. His colour therapy claimed much success. Further information can be obtained from the Spectrachrome Institute, Malaga, New Jersey. *See* Bibliography.
Dowsing	Very precise information about this practice is available from the British Society of Dowsers (*see Resources*).
The Egyptian Book of the Dead	It is known that the title has been wrongly translated and the symbols could also have meant 'The Egyptian Book of the Living'. It is actually a kind of instruction book, like the Old Testament or the Koran.
Electromagnetic spectrum	The range of all the vibrations that can be scientifically established, from very high cosmic rays (vibrations too fast for physical measurement) to very slow sound waves (7–14 cycles per second). Such low frequencies can actually destroy all biochemical structures.
Electronic ballast	In layman's terms, a converter which changes AC into DC, causing the electricity to become constant. It is used for fluorescent lights, stabilizing the gas used in the tubes and cutting out all flicker.
Fibonacci, Leonardo	(1175–1250). A Florentine mathematician who described the Fibonacci sequence of numbers. A contemporary of Francis of Assisi.
Fluorescent	A term used to describe the illumination issued by the gas-filled tubes which H. Heitler developed. The luminosity produced in certain substances also connected to X-rays and ultra-violet rays. *See also* Ott, John.
Francis, St	(1182–1226). A monk who lived in Assisi. The founder of the Franciscan order. He is probably among the best known saints of the Christian faith.

Galvanizer, skin	A sensitive instrument that records the tension of a person under certain environmental influences.
Geode	Stone with hollow cavities studded with crystals such as amethysts, quartz crystals and many other precious or semiprecious stones. Inside is also quite frequently found the still-liquid form of the growing crystals.
Glazewski, Dr Father Andrew	(1901–1973). A concert pianist and doctor of physics, he worked for nine years in the Vatican. He was also a great healer and studied Rudolf Steiner's anthroposophy.
Goethe, Johann Wolfgang von	(1749–1832). Scientist, poet and researcher, born in Frankfurt. *See* Bibliography.
Goetheanum	The school founded by Rudolf Steiner in 1911 in Dornach, Switzerland, to teach anthroposophy, a science to study man as part of the spiritual energies which stand behind all visible structures.
Gregory, Ronald	Professor of Psychology at Bristol University.
Gurdjieff, G.	Russian mystic. *See* Ouspensky (Bibliography).
Heitler, Dr Hans	(1899–1979). Physicist, expelled from Germany as a Jew. Worked under Professor Powell, Bristol University, in outer space research. Developed the first fluorescent tubes as emergency illumination.
Incandescent	The normal light bulbs which have a metallic filament absorbing about 70 per cent of electricity-producing heat and about 30 per cent of light.
König, Dr Karl	(1902–1966). Founder of the Campbell and Sheiling schools. Author and researcher.
Mantra	A sacred word or prayer that has the power to bring about physical and spiritual change when used as directed by a teacher or master.
Monochrome	Any item or object having only one colour of even hue.
The New Testament	A book containing the synoptic gospels and other teachings. It is known that other gospels existed which have not been published.
Newton, Sir Isaac	(1642–1727). Early English scientist who researched the natural phenomena of colour, gravity and their relationship to consciousness. *See* Bibliography.

The Old Testament	This book belongs to the teachings of the Jewish and Christian faiths. To some extent it is also part of the sacred teachings of the Moslems. All religions have their writings on human conduct and how to 'see' God. Through translations and the changes in human consciousness, many passages have been left out or not really understood.
Osiris	Egyptian god of the sun.
Ott, Dr John	Member of the Light and Health Research Council (MLHRC). The originator of the full-spectrum fluorescent tube. Researcher into children's learning capacity and into illumination. His contribution to interior illumination is world famous and very important.
Psyche	The Greek word for the human soul.
Spine	The divisions which constitute the spine are as follows: skull, cervical, thoracic, lumbar, sacrum and coccyx.
Steiner, Dr Rudolf	(1861–1925). Founder of the Anthroposophical Society in Dornach, Switzerland. He developed a spiritual science of the origin, make up and function of the human. Not a religious order.
Thoth	The Egyptian god of writing and the sciences and inventor of the arts, who kept a record of the actions of the dead.

Resources

Hygeia College of Colour Therapy

COLOUR HEALING COURSES

Northern Centre

4 Sunningdale Close

Kirkham

Preston

Lancashire

PR4 2TG

Tel: 01772 671128

Contact:

Jean & Tony Greenslade

London Centre

The School of Mantra Colour Healing

12 Rogers House

Page Street

London

SW1P 4EX

Tel: 0207 821 1143

Contact: Deborah Italiano

HYGEIA HEALTH PRODUCTS

Most of our products are made to order as all are hand-made. Contact Hygeia Studios at the Preston address above.

The Colour Space Illuminator

A lamp which can, at your own control, mix and change the illumination in your room for parties, meditation or relaxation.

The Hygeia Water Solarizer
An ancient method to induce colour into drinking water – for alertness or relaxation.

The Hygeia Visualization Cards
Eight colour-cards to refocus and relax your eyes after lengthy concentration working with VDUs, word processors, etc.

Eye Strengthening Chart
Two colours that have opposite polarity cause the eyes to 'breathe' and will enliven your sight.

The Eye Healing Lamp
With this lamp you can revitalize the eyes and combat glaucoma and cataracts. Regular use is vital but effective.

Colour Consciousness
Colour causes the stimulation of the right-brain functions. Form involves the left-brain activity. To unite the two halves arouses greater awareness.

The Colour Crystal Treatment Torch
('Co-crys-to') An instrument to balance the ductless gland system.

The Colour Crystal Lamp
A lamp which illuminates a crystal for healing purposes. A very sensitive energy can be induced into a clear quartz crystal used in conjunction with a set of full-spectrum filters (stained glass).

Full-Spectrum Stained Glass
Stained glass can be the most perfect filter to harmonize the human body.

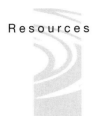

For full-spectrum glass:
Stephan Lamberts
Lamberts
Schützenstr. 1
Postfach 1106
D-95652 Waldsassen
Germany
Tel: +49 (0) 96 322371

For dowsing:
The British Society of Dowsers
Sycamore Barn
Hastingleigh
Ashford
Kent
TN25 5HW
Tel and Fax: (01233) 750253
www.britishdowsers.org
email: secretary@britishdowsers.org

Bibliography

Alpen, Dr Frank, *Exploring Atlantis*, Arizona Metaphysical Society, 1981.

Babbit, Edwin D., *The Principles of Light and Colour*, 1978.

Beesley, Ronald, *The Robe of Many Colours*, private publication, 1968.

— *The Creative Ether*, Neville Spearman, 1972.

Cade, Maxwell, *The Awakened Mind,* Element Books, 1989.

Critchlow, Keith, *Order in Space*, Thames & Hudson, 1969.

Dewhurst-Maddock, Olivia, *The Book of Sound Therapy*, Gaia, 1993.

Dinshah, P. Ghadiali, *Spectochrome Metry Encyclopaedia*, 3 vols., 1939.

Garde, Dr R. K., *Ayurveda for Health and Long Life*, D. B. Taraporevala Sons & Co. Private Ltd., India, 1975.

Gimbel, Theophilus, *Healing Through Colour*, C. W. Daniel, 1980.

— *Form, Sound, Colour and Healing*, C. W. Daniel, 1987.

— *Healing Colour*, Gaia Books, 2001

— *Sixteen Steps to Health and Energy*, Foulsham, 1992

— *Key, Lock and Door*, Hygeia College of Colour Therapy

— *The Power of the Third*, Hygeia College of Colour Therapy

— *Pythagoras: The Master Stories*, Hygeia College of Colour Therapy

Bibliography

— *The Healing Power of Colour*, Hygeia College of Colour Therapy

— *Colour: The Next Dimension of Healing*, Hygeia College of Colour Therapy

— *Art as a Medium for Healing*, Hygeia College of Colour Therapy

— Colour Consciousness, Hygeia College of Colour Therapy

Goethe, Johann Wolfgang von, *Die Farben Lehre* (The Teachings of Colour), 1810.

Haich, Elisabeth, *Initiation*, Mandala, 1979.

Hunt, Roland, *The Seven Keys to Colour Healing*, 11th edn, C. W. Daniel.

Kilian, J., *Crystals: Secrets of the Inorganic*, Scientific Book Club, 1940.

Kilner, Dr Walter John, *The Human Atmosphere* (orig. title, republished as *The Aura*), 1911.

Lüscher, Professor Max, *The Lüscher Colour Test*, Cape, 1969.

New Larousse Encyclopaedia of Mythology, Hamlyn, 1959.

Newton, Sir Isaac, *Philosophiae Naturalis Principia Mathematica*, 1687.

Ouseley, S. G. J., *The Power of the Rays*, L. N. Fowler, 1951.

Ouspensky, P. D., *In Search of the Miraculous*, Routledge Kegan Paul, 1949.

Pearl, Richard H., *Introduction to the Mineral Kingdom*, Blandford Press, London, 1966.

Prouskauer, Herrman, O., *Zum Studium von Goethes Farbenlehre*, Zbinden Verlag, Basel, 1968.

Silva, José, *Mind Control*, Simon & Schuster, 1977.

Thakkur, Dr Chandra Shekhar, G., *Ayurveda: The Science of Life*, ASI Publishers Inc., New York, 1974.

Tisserand, Robert B., *The Art of Aromatherapy*, C. W. Daniel, 1977.

Watson, Lyall, *Supernature*, Hodder & Stoughton, London, 1973.

Wills, Pauline, *The Reflexology and Colour Therapy Workbook*, Element, 1992.

— *Health Essentials: Colour Therapy*, Element, 1993.

Index

Index